DAD'S PREGNANT TOO!

TOO!

Expectant fathers, expectant mothers, new dads, and new moms share **advice, tips, and stories about all the surprises, questions, and joys ahead…**

Harlan Cohen

SOURCEB____, INC.
NAPERVILLE, ILLINOIS

© 2008 by Harlan Cohen
Cover and internal design © 2008 by Sourcebooks, Inc.
Cover design by Cyanotype Book Architects
Cover image © Veer
Images in Chapter 3 © 2008 A.D.A.M., Inc.

Sourcebooks and the colophon are registered trademarks of Sourcebooks, Inc.

All rights reserved. No part of this book may be reproduced in any form or by any electronic or mechanical means including information storage and retrieval systems—except in the case of brief quotations embodied in critical articles or reviews—without permission in writing from its publisher, Sourcebooks, Inc.

This book is not intended as a substitute for medical advice from a qualified physician. The intent of this book is to provide accurate general information in regard to the subject matter covered. If medical advice or other expert help is needed, the services of an appropriate medical professional should be sought.

All brand names and product names used in this book are trademarks, registered trademarks, or trade names of their respective holders. Sourcebooks, Inc., is not associated with any product or vendor in this book.

Published by Sourcebooks, Inc.
P.O. Box 4410, Naperville, Illinois 60567-4410
(630) 961-3900
Fax: (630) 961-2168
www.sourcebooks.com

Library of Congress Cataloging-in-Publication Data
Cohen, Harlan
   Dad's pregnant too : expectant fathers, expectant mothers, new dads, and new moms share advice, tips, and stories about all the surprises, questions, and joys ahead / Harlan Cohen.
      p. cm.
   Includes bibliographical references and index.
   1. Pregnancy—Popular works. 2. Childbirth—Popular works.
3. Fatherhood. 4. Husbands. I. Title.
   RG525.C658 2008
   618.2—dc22

                              2008014818

Printed and bound in the United States of America.
VP 10 9 8 7 6 5 4 3 2 1

It all started on 3/2/01 – it was the night of our first date when we started this fun.

And now, the journey continues…

I love you.

To Stephanie, EKC & Happy Ha Ha

THANK YOU FOR HELPING ME GIVE BIRTH...

I'd like to thank Stephanie, my pregnant wife/best friend/inspiration/partner/love of my life. Thank you for letting me test my theories and hypotheses on you during this pregnancy. You are the most beautiful pregnant woman in the world. In fact, from behind, you don't even look pregnant. I'd like to thank my daughter Eva Kaye (Harlephanie was her prenatal name). Thank you for being so well-behaved in the womb (and outside). You are the greatest gift in the world and we love you so much (p.s. if we mess up, let us know and we'll make things better or get you the best therapy available). Thank you to my mom (Shirlee) and dad (Eugene) for creating me and to my mom for giving birth to me. In fact, I'd like to take this opportunity to formally apologize to you, Mom. Sorry I was two weeks overdue and that I had to be delivered via a surprise C-section. I don't know what I was thinking—if I could do it all over again I'd have popped out at 7 $\frac{1}{2}$ pounds and saved you the hassle (and scar). Please accept my apology. I love you. And thank you Dad for being the best father in the world. While you didn't get a chance to cut the cord because you weren't invited into the delivery room (I'll find you some kind of cord to cut later if you want), I love you as much as a son can love his dad. Thank you to my brothers Vic and Michael, and my sister-in-law Irene—your advice, guidance, help, love, hand-me downs, and breast pump were so deeply appreciated (clarification—the breast pump was from Irene). Thank you to my nieces Phoebe and Rae and my nephew Henry. You have been the cutest and best practice babies for Steph and me. I'd like to thank my in-laws Fran, Marvin, Dan, and Rozi. Fran and Marvin, I think that if you could have given birth to me you would have done it, but instead, you gave birth to my wife—and that's more than enough for me. Your constant love, support, and encouragement are deeply appreciated. A heartfelt thank you goes out to friends, family, and all the random contributors I accosted while researching this book. Thank you for opening up your lives and sharing your most personal, emotional, embarrassing, and deeply honest stories as part of this book. Your experiences are what make this project so compelling. Thank you to all the doctors, nurses, and caregivers who helped us through pregnancy, labor, and delivery and the pregnancy, labor, and delivery of this book. My deepest gratitude goes out to my long time editorial obstetrician, Peter Lynch (please do not edit this Peter). You are a gifted handler of thoughts, ideas, and words—thank you for helping me push and deliver this book from my womb (again, no editing). Thanks to Todd Stocke (director of editorial obstetrics), and the editorial, sales, publicity, and support teams at Sourcebooks. A heartfelt thank you goes out to Dominique Raccah, chief editorial obstetrician (Sourcebook's publisher). Your passion, commitment, and encouragement are an inspiration. A thank you goes out to my agent/midwife, Eliot Ephraim. You continue to be right there by my side throughout the personal and professional journey. Thank you to Glenn Mott and the entire team at King Features Syndicate, the newspaper editors who have supported my Help Me, Harlan! syndicated advice column over the years, the readers of Help Me, Harlan!, the students and professionals who have invited me to share my passion on college campuses over the years, The Indiana University School of Journalism, the Indiana Daily Student, and the late Dr. Dave Adams (still can't believe you're gone—I miss you).

Finally, thank you to the readers of this book. It's a privilege to have the opportunity to share this experience and time with you. I look forward to what I hope will be the beginning of a long relationship with you as you experience the most amazing, profound, surreal, and awesome adventure of your life.

Thank you,
Harlan Cohen

CONTENTS

Chapter 1
The First Few Weeks…
Shock, Joy, Surprise, and Things
You'll Want to Do

Chapter 2
The Doctor Will See You Now
Or Whoever Delivers Your Baby
Will See You Now

Chapter 3

The Baby's Development

Chapter 4

The Many Faces of the Expectant Father

Chapter 7

Spoiling Your Pregnant Partner

Chapter 8

Pregnant Sex

Having It, Not Having It, Fantasizing

Chapter 12

The Birth Day

From Your Door to Delivery Room and

Chapter 13

After the Baby is Born

THE CONCEPTION

HOW IT HAPPENED...

It might have happened on your honeymoon, on vacation, on a first date, in an elevator, on an escalator, on the bathroom floor, on the kitchen counter, in the bedroom, after senior prom, at a friend's wedding, at your own wedding, in a doctor's office, at a fertility clinic, with the help of a surrogate, or through an adoption agency. It might have happened on purpose, by accident, or by chance. It could have been a broken condom, a missed pill, a romantic evening, a one night stand, a fluke, or a well-orchestrated plan involving ovulation kits and basal thermometers. You might have been trying for minutes, days, weeks, months, or years. You might be single. You might be married. You might be separated. You might be in love, in lust, in like, or neither. The news might be shocking, scary, exciting, overwhelming, or not *real* considering not much has changed (assuming you're in the first trimester). How it happened, when it happened, where it happened, or why it happened is all in the past. All that matters is that it's happened. What you will encounter next is *the most* exhilarating, emotional, intense, intimidating, and awesome experience of your entire life.

Congratulations!

The following pages will offer a never-before-seen look into the expectant father experience. It's everything a dad-to-be can expect to see, hear, feel, touch, taste, and smell (see Tip #36).

Never before in the history of men and women have expectant fathers been so involved in the pregnancy process. From conception to delivery, we are attending appointments, holding legs, helping her push, positioning mirrors, cutting cords, changing diapers, taking care of our partners, taking care of the baby, and doing it all. While women expect us to be more involved and helpful than ever before, there's so little information to help us know what to do and how to do it. While women have hundreds of years of oral and written history handed down from generation to generation, today's expectant fathers are the first generation living in this unprecedented time in history. Other than our friends telling us over and over again, "You have no idea how life will change, man" we have little more to go on.

But now, that's all about to change…

Dad's Pregnant Too is a living piece of work that will grow over time. If you have a resource that's helped you, send it my way. If you have a story, advice, or tip— send it over. Email me at Harlan@helpmeharlan.com or Harlan@dadspregnant.com. You can also submit your stories and tips via www.DadsPregnant.com. Also, please check out the Dad's Pregnant online forums and Facebook Fan page.

Again, thank you for picking up this book. I look forward to sharing this experience with you. Enjoy the adventure…it's a wild ride.

Thank you,
Harlan Cohen

WELCOME EXPECTANT FATHERS

As a two-time expectant father, I can appreciate that the last thing a lot of guys want to do is read a book for expectant fathers. I promise not to waste your time.

If you were reading this book 35 years ago, it would be a few pages and simple. Get her pregnant, go to work, sit in the waiting room, celebrate, go home, and go back to work. But in the past 35 years, things have dramatically changed. We are now as close to the action as a man can possibly get. We see it, hear it, feel it, smell it, and even touch it (flip to Tip #33, but don't touch without her permission).

From the first GUYne visit to holding her leg while she pushes to catching a glimpse of her BV (birthing vagina) to holding the baby for the first time following a C-section, we are truly pioneers. Women expect us to do more because we have never been more involved. On top of everything that's happening with our partner and the baby, we're dealing with so many changes and new feelings on so many levels. It's normal to feel overwhelmed at times.

As I interviewed hundreds of men and women, it became clear to me this project was much bigger than I had ever imagined. As you will read in the pages to follow, we are treading in unchartered amniotic waters. We are the first generation in thousands of years to play this role. It's no wonder we don't always know what the hell is happening—when you're the first it's hard to take it all in. Up to now, what we can expect as an expectant father has largely been a mystery. And really, dramatic change + no answers + little information = a stressful experience.

The information on the pages to follow will enable expectant fathers to see what's coming their way so they can get comfortable with the uncomfortable. While each and every one of these situations might not play out for you, a majority of them will. Simply knowing what's coming your way (even if you can't change it) can help you face the experience with greater confidence, clarity, and control.

And that's what this is all about.

As you page through this book, consider using it to help you stay connected with your pregnant partner. Use it to your advantage. For example, when attempting to have sex with your pregnant partner, flip to Tip #57 and bounce the seduction techniques off her. Ask her to pick the one that will work. If she starts freaking out and getting scared about having a baby, Tip #47 will remind her that being scared is normal. Read her the tip and story. If you feel like she's in a bad place emotionally, check out the depression Tip #49 and ask her about some of the warning signs.

One more thing worth mentioning: I've included pictures in this book (see Chapter 3). No other book I've seen for men offers a detailed week by week development of the baby. Men are visual, and it helps to see it all happen. Check out these pages and stay involved and up to date with the pregnancy. While she has 40 weeks to feel pregnant, we have to work to find ways to stay connected and engaged. I hope the images and information help.

As I mentioned in the intro, this is the first edition of what will be many to come. If something rubs you the wrong way, please let me know. If there is a resource that's helped you, send it my way. If you have a story, advice, or tip—please send it over. You can email me at Harlan@helpmeharlan.com or Harlan@dadspregnant.com. You can also submit stories and tips via www.DadsPregnant.com and contribute to the expectant forums online at www.DadsPregnant.com. And if you're on Facebook, please check out the Dad's Pregnant Too Facebook group.

Thanks again,
Harlan

WELCOME EXPECTANT MOTHERS

First, thanks for not making us carry the baby. I'm still completely blown away by what your body does and how well you are able to manage it. I'm not kissing your butt (well, maybe a little); I genuinely feel this way. The female body is awesome. Creating life, carrying it for 40 weeks (or so), and then having to get it out of your body is something I can't even imagine, because unless you've lived it, there's no way to understand it.

While you're going through the most dramatic physical and emotional changes of your life, we are supposed to be there for you. We are supposed to say the right things and do the right things. We are supposed to take care of you and ourselves and be cool the whole time it's happening. The reality is that we are dealing with our own changes. We want to be supportive, and we want to be helpful (at least most of us), but it's hard to know what to do or how to do it being that this is the first time we're dealing with it too.

While there are countless books for women dealing with pregnancy, there isn't one I've seen that focuses on the role of men and what women wish their partners would do to help make this experience more comfortable both physically and emotionally. That's what this book is about.

While interviewing women for this project, I'd ask them what their partners did right, what they did wrong, and what they could do better. Not only can you read the answers that other women have shared, the information should give you a little bit of insight into what your partner is feeling and how to help him better understand what you're going through.

As I've mentioned earlier, this is the first edition of many editions to follow. I'm sure there are many more issues, stories, and tips that should be included to help men get it right the first time. Please share your expert advice. If there are things you'd like to see in future editions, let me know. If there are things you'd like me to get rid of in future editions, let me know. You can email me at Harlan@helpmeharlan.com or Harlan@ dadspregnant.com. You can also submit stories and tips via www.DadsPregnant.com and contribute to the expectant forums online at www.DadsPregnant.com. And if you're on Facebook, please check out the Dad's Pregnant Too Facebook group.

Thank you,
Harlan

WELCOME HEALTH PROFESSIONALS

First, I'd like to start by thanking you for the work you do. With so many different personality types walking in and out of your offices and everyone's emotions running high (not to mention the premiums for insurance running high) it must be as thrilling as it is exhausting to do what you do on a daily basis. I can't imagine a more rewarding or demanding job than bringing new life into the world on a daily basis.

As an expectant father who attended every prenatal appointment and talked to hundreds of parents who went through the same process, I have a much deeper appreciation of what it means to receive care when going through this experience. I hope this book can become an invaluable resource to help expectant men and women get comfortable with a naturally uncomfortable experience. I hope it will encourage them to ask questions freely, share their concerns, and feel more connected to their caregivers.

I did my very best to provide a balanced point of view. I made a concerted effort to avoid advocating one practice over another. I advocate patient education so that each individual can make an informed decision that's aligned with their values. I know this experience is a deeply personal and emotional one for patients and caregivers. If you come across something in this book that can be improved or better balanced, let me know. Likewise, if you love something, please let me know.

As I mentioned earlier, I like to think of this book as a living breathing work (but you will not find a pulse using your Doppler). Please share any feedback you can offer. I would be thrilled to consider including your stories and tips (always anonymous) in future editions. Please email me at Harlan@helpmeharlan.com or via Harlan@dadspregnant.com. You can also submit stories and tips via www.DadsPregnant.com and contribute to the expectant forums online at www.DadsPregnant.com. And if you're on Facebook, please check out the Dad's Pregnant Too Facebook group.

Thank you!
Harlan

HOW THIS BOOK WAS PUT TOGETHER

As a syndicated advice columnist for the past twelve years, people have been sharing their deepest secrets with me for my entire adult life. My favorite part of my advice column is sharing stories from people who have been there and lived it. It's the people who are living it or have recently lived it who are some of the most credible experts.

This book captures the voices of these experts—it's people who have lived it or have recently lived it sharing their tips, stories, and insight. As you go through your experience, I hope you will share your stories and insight as it unfolds. My goal is to provide the most complete look at the expectant father experience.

HOW THIS BOOK WAS RESEARCHED

- I GOT SOMEONE PREGNANT. Actually, we kind of planned it, so it worked out well. She was receptive to the idea. She had never been pregnant, and I had never gotten a woman pregnant, so it was all a new experience. My experience is central to this, but I'm just one of the guys who has been there and done it.
- I GOT SOMEONE PREGNANT AGAIN. Again, we kind of planned it so it made the process easier. Going through the experience for a second time while writing this book was surreal. Having a little distance from the first experience and seeing how it unfolded the second time

around helped to provide some clarity and put things in perspective.

- I INTERVIEWED EXPECTANT AND NEW DADS. I talked to hundreds of expectant dads. I posted requests online, spoke to people over the phone, and talked to people face to face. I asked them to share their tips and the stories behind the tips. Tips are suggestions lacking context—the stories behind the tip are where the real wisdom can be gleaned.
- I INTERVIEWED EXPECANT AND NEW MOMS. This was tricky. I would stop women who looked pregnant and talk to them. If I wasn't sure they were pregnant, I would just tell them I needed directions after stopping them and realizing, "Oh crap! I can't tell if you're really pregnant." Interviews were conducted face-to-face, online, over the phone, in airports, at malls, in coffee shops, and wherever else I saw a big belly or stroller headed my way.
- I INTERVIEWED MEDICAL EXPERTS. One of my favorite questions I'd ask the doctors when researching the book was, "What *can't* you say to a patient, but you've always wanted to say…" I felt it was important to talk to doctors so that the information in this book would be accurate and helpful.
- I REVIEWED RELEVANT MATERIALS. If you walked into my office you would think that I'm either a little too excited about having

another baby or writing a book. Anything I could get my hands on, I would read. One of the coolest things was getting daily Google Alerts. You can sign up for alerts at Google and then get stories from around the world that include relevant keywords you've submitted. Every morning I read about the news with the keywords "Expectant Father" and "Pregnant Woman."

WHAT MAKES THIS BOOK UNIQUE

I remember telling some people I was writing a book about pregnancy, and they were like, "There are so many out there…Are you crazy?" Their point was that everything had already been said. But as I dug deeper into the issues, it became obvious to me that there was a huge gaping hole when it came to books dealing with men and the way couples interact when going through the pregnancy experience. Most women's pregnancy books either talk about what's happening with their bodies or the baby's body. There are a select few that address the mind and body experience, but even those are written from a woman's point of view. When it comes to books for guys, the biggest problem is that there aren't a lot of them. As the first generation of men in the delivery room, few of us have had a chance to live it and digest it—let alone write about it.

Almost every guy I spoke with told me he would take his partner's pregnancy books and look at the pictures of the baby's development (makes sense, guys are visual). So, I wanted to give guys some pictures (you'll find those on pages 83–101). Another thing men would mention is that they would often say or do the wrong thing by accident. They would try their hardest only to end up looking like an accidental asshole. To help guys gain better insight into the experience and reduce their risks of turning into an accidental asshole, I felt it was important for women to directly address men so we could get a better understanding of what they're feeling and thinking (a lot of women who are pregnant can't express it because it's all so new). Lastly, men don't talk to men about their fears and insecurities all that often. We all have them, but few share them. To address this, I asked men to share the things they've never told anyone else—their fears, frustrations, and most intimate and revealing moments. The composite should help men get a better sense of the changes and challenges coming their way and enable women to better understand the changes happening in the lives of their partners. The goal is to make the experience less about fearing the unknown and more about coming together as a couple and managing whatever comes your way.

ABOUT THE TIPS AND STORIES

As you flip through the pages, you'll read a tip and a story. The majority of the stories you'll read are verbatim, from the mouths of the people sharing them. Some tips and stories were submitted via my website (www.HelpMeHarlan.com) and others were gathered via interviews. If I interviewed someone and didn't have a pad and paper, I would later write the stories down in the voice of the person relaying the story. When attributing stories, I used the name of the person sharing the story and the age and gender or genders of that person's child or children. A small percentage of the contributors asked me to change their first name to protect their identity. If a tip or story was submitted using an alias, I would assign a name to the story submitted. The goal was to create a free flowing dialogue where people could share *whatever* was on their minds. I've found that this method of sharing is successful in allowing contributors to feel completely at ease.

ABOUT THE CONTENT AND WORD CHOICES

In writing this book I conducted a tremendous amount of research. Along the way, I would discover that some people have *very* passionate opinions about how to navigate this experience. I included information about natural birth, home birth, hospital birth, doulas, midwives, doctors, epidural, no pain medication, nursing, formula feeding, and other issues about which people have very strong beliefs. I did my very best to offer a balanced view of the expectant father experience. This book isn't about me forcing any one belief or practice on an individual, but reporting the experience in a manner that shows all differing points of view. I avoided using the words "husbands" and "wives" and instead used "partners." I often used the word "caregiver" instead of "doctor." I frequently used "birth location" instead of "hospital." If you have a particular point of view, and would like me to consider it for future editions, please send it to me by emailing me at Harlan@helpmeharlan.com or via www.DadsPregnant.com. I know this is a sensitive area and want to make sure all sides and all voices are represented.

NOPE, THIS ISN'T A MEDICAL GUIDE

While conducting research I interviewed medical professionals, included trusted and medically reviewed content, and this book has been medically reviewed. That said, I am not a doctor. This book is not a medical guide. If you have questions, please consult your caregiver. This book may help you to come up with questions and be more comfortable asking questions, but any concerns you have should be addressed by a medical professional.

THE FIRST OF MANY EDITIONS

If you've read this whole intro you're probably getting tired of me telling you that this is a living, breathing piece of work (it's not actually living and breathing—it's a book). The plan is to update this book frequently to include the latest information, facts, stats, and insight. Your experiences and your stories are crucial to this process. If you're familiar with my bestselling book on college life (*The Naked Roommate: and 107 Other Issues You Might Run Into in College*) you'll know that your voices are the most important part of this experience. I'm just the one putting the pieces together.

I ask that you please share with me your thoughts and feelings. If you like something, let me know. If you don't like something, let me know. If there's something missing in here, please let me know. If you think I've gotten something wrong, let me know. You can swear at me and call me names, but please make sure there's a suggestion after you're done berating me. Please email me at Harlan@helpmeharlan.com or via Harlan@dadspregnant.com or via www.Dads Pregnant.com. Thank you so much for the support. I look forward to hearing from you.

WE ARE PIONEERS...

Two weeks after her due date, my mom checked into the hospital to have me. She was given a bed in labor and delivery, my dad was given a chair in the expectant fathers' waiting room. There was no holding her hand, comforting her through labor, encouraging her to push, hearing the baby's first cry, cutting the cord, or documenting the first moments of my life. He was told to wait outside the door.

Fast forward thirty-five years and the door has swung wide open.

We are no longer stuck in the waiting room; we are in the trenches watching it unfold in real time. We are holding her hand, helping her push, cutting the cord, seeing it, hearing it, and experiencing it all. We have a front row seat. We see it, feel it, and hear about it like no man of our parents' generation has seen, heard, or felt it. From conception to homecoming, we are true pregnancy pioneers. Unlike the sisterhood of women who have been sharing pregnancy stories and offering guidance through the ages, up until now, men have had few resources. But now, that's all about to change....

1

THE FIRST FEW WEEKS...

Shock, Joy, Surprise, and Things You'll Want to Do

Tip #1
THE MAGIC URINE: The Day We Officially Lose Control

THE TIP:
You can take a pregnancy test yourself, but only hers counts.

THE STORY:
The first four tests she took were all positive, but the indicator strips were extremely light. That's when I took a fifth test to act as a control test to make sure the results were accurate. She laughed at first but generally thought I was an idiot for doing so. She stood next

to me as I took the test (she turned away when I peed). After dipping the stick, my wife watched as the indicator light revealed the results. As predicted, the results were a bright negative. For some reason, I had to test it. I just couldn't believe it.

—Scott, daughter 23 months

* * *

The lack of control begins with her urine.

My wife hoarded her pee—she insisted it was too early to take a pregnancy test and refused to pee on a stick for me. I insisted that even though it was too early, taking a pregnancy test is too much fun to pass up. How many times in our life do we get to do this?

I like to think of taking a pregnancy test like being on a game show without the game show music in the background (although next time I think I might play music during the test). The prize is that you get to have a baby (or two or three). I explained to her that it wasn't fair that she was hoarding her urine. She then explained that she didn't want to be disappointed if the test was negative like the previous month's round of testing.

After explaining to her that a negative result is the most likely result, and that it would be too soon to be disappointed because it's so early, she yielded and reluctantly offered me some of her possibly pregnant urine. She then dipped the pregnancy test stick and we huddled around the urine-soaked magic wand.

Pregnancy tests work by detecting the pregnancy hormone hCG. HCG begins to be produced when a fertilized egg implants in the uterus—about 6 days after conception—and then continues to increase during pregnancy. Most pregnancy tests give the most accurate results once hCG reaches high enough levels in the urine to be detected, about one week after a missed period. Early pregnancy tests can be used to tell if you're pregnant up to five days before a missed period.

Once we dipped the stick and waited two minutes, we saw what appeared to be the faintest blue line. I bought a cheap test because…I can be cheap at times. The line was so faint it almost wasn't there. It definitely wasn't negative, but it was barely positive. We angled it, we put it under a bright light, dipped it in the urine cup on the counter—still, we thought the results were unclear.

I then peed on one of the sticks to see if they were defective (surprisingly a number of guys do this). Fast forward 15 minutes, and I returned home from the drugstore with three deluxe digital home pregnancy tests. She peed again, we huddled again, and then, the word *pregnant* flashed on the screen. We took another test and it said *not pregnant*. She then took another digital test from a different manufacturer, and the results flashed *pregnant*. We figured two flashing pregnant sticks meant that she was really pregnant.

I've heard that tests *rarely* ever give false positives. (hCG levels can vary from day to day, which can make someone have a positive test one day, and then a

PREGNANCY Q & A:

QUESTION: Number of pregnancy tests she took?
ANSWER: Around three or four.

QUESTION: How long it took for her to get pregnant?
ANSWER: About two months.

QUESTION: Where it happened (location)?
ANSWER: We think conception happened at home on the middle landing of the (carpeted) stairs the night after we saw the movie *The Break Up*.

negative test the next.) So a positive result normally means that you can be pretty sure she is pregnant. My wife took another test with her morning pee, and we were 100 percent positive. Four cheap tests and three digital tests later (a total of $75 worth of sticks), we finally believed she was pregnant.

So much of pregnancy is about facing the unknown and accepting your lack of control. As a man, we don't even have control over the test—that's how little control we have from day one. But if you accept this fact and embrace the reality that you will experience an incredible amount of surprise during pregnancy—some surprises difficult, but most extremely good—you quickly learn how to get comfortable with the uncomfortable right from the start.

THE BOTTOM LINE:

Put your urine away and go with her flow. There's no controlling the future even if you pee on a control stick.

THE TIP:

The first few days are surreal; then normal life returns.

THE STORY:

We had been trying to get pregnant for eight months. The lack of control we had over our ability to conceive was a source of discomfort. The longer we tried, the more impatient we started to feel. By month four of trying to conceive, we knew we were doing everything in our power to become pregnant and that some of this process was just out of our control, so we started to release ourselves to the universe. We also switched from the pregnancy test with the lines to the test that had a smiley face as the positive indicator (the marketing got us—what would you rather see, a line or a smile?). This particular morning we were both standing around the bathroom sink waiting for the test to reveal the answer. When the smiley face began to emerge, we just stared at it in disbelief. We gave it a couple of more minutes to turn negative, but it stayed positive. We couldn't believe it worked. Once the disbelief subsided, there was happiness, then a fear that it wouldn't stick (some of our friends had miscarried), then excitement that it happened, followed by relief that we could conceive. It's funny, the month we got pregnant was the month we relied on the least amount of science to get pregnant.

—Mike, son 3 months

✳ ✳ ✳

The moment you hear the news, you go from man to expectant father. The emotions are wild and can include disbelief, shock, happiness, surprise, fear, joy, disappointment, relief, panic (financial worries), victory, regret, pride, guilt, ecstasy, and numbness.

Once the initial shock and emotions wane, things get quiet. Other than the pregnancy test, her sore boobs, exhaustion, nausea, and a pile of pregnancy books scattered around the house, not much has changed. You wake up for work, do your job, and then come home. You know something big is happening, but there's not a lot of visual evidence to support this monumental change. You go from experiencing a surreal moment of mind-blowing craziness, elation, and fear to passing the time.

In the meantime, she might not even feel like she's pregnant, but emotionally she knows she's pregnant. But men are programmed very differently than women. Men are visual creatures (see Tip #59). Until we can see it, touch it, or hear it, we have a hard time processing it. We need to see that ultrasound, to hear that heartbeat, to touch her big belly, or to have some

He found out Christmas morning. I put the pregnancy test in his stocking. He kept looking at me confused and surprised, saying, "Really?"
—Cathy (sons 4 months, 3½ years)

kind of tactile evidence, other than a faint plus sign on a stick, to grab onto the fact that things are changing. It can take months for it to hit you. I'm convinced that pregnancy lasts so long because it takes a guy a good five months to believe it (and another four months to get the furniture delivered).

On the other side of the bed is a first-time expectant mother consumed with the unknown. All her energy goes into the pregnancy from the moment the test turns positive. She'll go online and find a pregnancy pal. She might add a due date tracker to the bottom of her email messages. She'll buy pregnancy books (she might have picked this one up for you). She'll subscribe to pregnancy magazines, order catalogs (for the baby's room), shop for maternity clothing, register for baby stuff, clean the house, and do anything else that can help her start preparing for the big event.

In the meantime, a man's life barely changes. He just has to do some things he might not want to do (shop, clean, listen, run errands). It's a similar experience to what happens when a woman gets engaged. The moment the ring goes on her finger she's off to the races planning the wedding. It's total immersion—books, magazines, planners, conversations with friends, and anything else she can consume to help her with what's

We had just returned from a week's vacation and pretty much knew we were preggers, and it was *very* unplanned. I just came out of the bathroom that morning crying and holding a very positive test stick. After I crawled back into the bed next to him, he said, "I've never been so scared, excited, and proud all at the same time…My boys can swim!!!"

—*Misti (daughter 24 months)*

next. When a guy sees his bride walking down the aisle, that's when he starts to get excited because he knows that it's real. It's not that we don't care. We're just programmed differently.

The challenge here is that a woman might misinterpret our actions (or lack thereof) as uncaring. She might think that we're not as happy if we're not doing as much as she is to get ready for the baby. So the best way to connect is to take an active role. She won't force you—you have to be willing and proactive.

One way to be involved is to read the week-by-week pregnancy developments during the first week or two after you find out. (This section is something you won't find in any other expectant father book.) The first 12 weeks of pregnancy are some of the most crucial, remarkable, and dramatic weeks of development. While you can't see what's happening by looking at her, you can see what's happening by looking at the section in this book about the baby's growth. If you follow what's going on, you can't help but be drawn into the experience. You'll find yourself getting excited. When you get excited, you won't have to work so hard to convince her that you're part of this process.

Keeping up with the pregnancy and taking an active role will help you stay connected and involved. If she knows you're there for her, this whole experience will be easier for her. It all starts during the first weeks, when the only sign she's pregnant is the indicator stick, her increased appetite, and that weird sense in your gut that something big is coming.

THE BOTTOM LINE:

Since they don't have a camera inside the uterus to broadcast the action, you have to take an active role to find out what's happening. Check out pages 83–101 for a week-by-week guide to what's happening inside (yes, there are pictures).

Tip #3
SHARING THE NEWS: Who, When, and How to Tell

THE TIP:

When you're not yet telling people and someone asks, it's really hard to lie about it.

THE STORY:

Our agreement was that if somebody asked, then we would tell. When somebody asks if you are pregnant, and you are, you can't help but hesitate, and they know if you say no that you're lying. So we had planned to tell our family first at Thanksgiving. My wife has a close group of grade school friends, and one of them had a baby shower. The whole time, she dodged the topic. She even snuck in a glass of orange juice while everybody else was drinking mimosas. Finally as it was time to leave, some random coworker of the hostess approaches my wife and blurts out, "I noticed you weren't drinking. Are you pregnant?" The secret was out. My parents flew in for Thanksgiving, and we had everybody over for dinner. Before we ate, I gave a toast to thank God for all his blessings over the past year. I closed the prayer by asking God to watch over us as we welcome the newest member of our family next July. After a couple of seconds, everybody understood what I was trying to say and lots of noise and congrats followed. My usually nonemotional father even started to tear up.

—Kevin, 3 months pregnant

* * *

Finding out that you're going to have a baby is a big moment and it's natural to want to tell the world. But most experts recommend waiting to share, which can be difficult and frustrating. Carrying around the biggest secret of your life is hard. What makes it even harder for a guy is that telling people makes it real. It helps to hear the words, "We're expecting."

The only problem is that telling too soon or too many people can cause problems. The decision about who and when to tell is completely different for each couple, but here are some things to consider before sending out a blast email and letting friends, family, and coworkers know the exciting news. (I know, it's so tempting to let everyone know.)

There are so many celebratory events that occur in your life that you tell everyone. This one was so uniquely special because it was a secret between us.
—Don (sons 22 months and 4 months)

WHY WAIT?

A lot of people will wait until 12 weeks into the pregnancy to share the news with the world. After the 12-week checkup, the chances of miscarriage go down. Telling before 12 weeks means that if the pregnancy should end, you'll have to explain to all the people who received your blast email that you are no longer expecting. And this personal process isn't something everyone wants to share publicly. Waiting to tell protects you from having to explain yourself should something not go as planned.

If your pregnant partner wants to tell more people than you originally agreed to tell, don't be so quick to limit her or make her feel bad for sharing. She might need more support than she thought she would need. Just make sure she tells you who she tells. This way, if she tells a friend and that friend tells your friend, you will know that your friend knows, and you won't have to lie if he asks you about it. Assume that if she tells her friend, that friend will tell her significant other, even if she forbids her from telling (no one can keep it a secret).

WHY WAIT?

Not all employers react as favorably as you might hope to an employee having a baby. Once you tell, word will travel fast. The reality is that having a baby can be disruptive to work (especially for

With one of our pregnancies we told too soon, and it unfortunately ended in a miscarriage. Waiting until after the first trimester is always recommended—now we know why. It saves a whole lot of heartache that can happen if people still think you're pregnant and you aren't anymore.

—*Patrick (father of 5, expecting #6)*

women). There's something to be said about waiting and telling employers until you have to let them know. Having your significant other tell them early doesn't do anything other than cause her boss to start wondering right away what is going to happen to her desire to work after she gives birth.

WHY WAIT?

Some people are superstitious. They think that telling will affect the pregnancy. I don't believe that superstition will change the outcome, although I'm not going to commit to this (call me superstitious). What's so interesting about superstition is that these rules we live by have no rational foundation. But, when dealing with the unknown and having so little control over the process, we tend to make rules. So, in a way, superstitions are just about control. That's one reason you'll find so many people are so superstitious when it comes to having a baby.

THE ODD RESPONSE

Some people will respond to the news with an odd response. Expect it. For example, childhood friends, single and unattached friends, jealous siblings, parents, and crazy relatives often say idiotic things. For example, you say, "I've got some exciting news. WE'RE EXPECTING A BABY!!!" And they may respond with:
- "Why? Why? Why?"
- "You're happy about this?"

- "You, a dad? No way!"
- "You're so screwed!"
- "I should have let you borrow that condom."
- "So, you keeping it?"
- "What the hell are you thinking?"
- "Does she know?"
- "Are you sure it's yours?"
- "I didn't even know you had sex!"
- "You're such a dumbass!"

Expect some stupid, weird, and confusing comments. Everyone gets them.

As a first-time expectant father, any feedback other than the feedback you expect to get can put you on the defensive or on the attack (you really might get pissed). Recognize that the reactions are more about them than you. For example, the news might make a childhood friend feel threatened, a parent feel old (as they realize that they are going to be a grandma or grandpa), a single sibling feel jealous, or a boss concerned. Their reactions aren't always about you or your parenting skills. If someone says something that bothers you, calmly tell them their response makes you uncomfortable ("uncomfortable" is a powerful nonconfrontational word that says it all). At least this way they can explain, and you can give them the chance not to be stupid twice.

THE BOTTOM LINE:
Share the news, but don't expect everyone to respond how you want them to respond. Some people, whether they mean to or not, will make stupid comments.

THE TIP:
We used a midwife for both pregnancies. If I hadn't had a vasectomy, we'd use one again.

THE STORY:
The midwife was already part of my wife's gynecologist's office, so it just worked out. I didn't know what a midwife did, but my wife filled me in. Some appointments were with the doctor and some were with the midwife. Both of them were good about asking us how we were doing. There were only two professionals in the practice so I got to know everyone, even the secretary. (I went to all the appointments.) It was a small and friendly place. The midwife was kind of a mentor during the pregnancy and delivery. She would ask me what I wanted to do and then offer me instructions. When my wife, who wanted to have a natural delivery (no medication), had to get an epidural and Pitocin because her labor was not moving along, the midwife was there to reassure us. We used the same doctor and midwife for our second baby.

—*Jim, daughter 2 months, son 3¼ years*

✻✻✻

Some doctors can have a more clinical and "just the facts" style. Our midwife answered all the questions and took time with us at each appointment.
—*Mike (son 12 months)*

While you might be an expert in getting the baby inside her, you need experts who can get the baby out of her. Different caregivers have different styles, approaches, and areas of expertise. Also, where she decides to give birth and the method she chooses will have an impact on who delivers. While physician-assisted births are the most common scenario, someone opting for a natural (nonmedicated) birth in a hospital or birthing center might want to have a midwife or doula present for labor and delivery. If you don't know what a midwife or doula is, you're like most of us (I'll explain it in a second).

If your partner is interested in bringing a doula or midwife into the equation, talk to men who have been there and done it. What you'll discover is that a midwife or doula isn't interested in stealing the spotlight. Your role and your participation will be part of the birth plan (as long as you want it to be part of the plan).

If working with an ob/gyn, have your partner ask the doctor how he or she feels about having a doula or midwife participating in labor and delivery. Again, some doctors may have strong reactions (pro or con). It helps to know how the ob/gyn feels about having someone else involved in the procedure before delivery so there won't be any surprises. Some ob/gyns might have a relationship with someone he or she can recommend. On the other hand, your partner might discover that her doctor might not want a doula assisting—finding this out on the day of the delivery is not a good thing. If you feel strongly about having one, then you will be faced with a decision about whether or not this is the right doctor for you. What matters the most is that your partner is comfortable and that you can talk freely to members of the team—whomever they may be.

THE DOCTOR
Talking to her regular ob/gyn is the natural place to begin. If you're thinking about a natural delivery or birth outside of the hospital, a family physician might be the right fit. Sometimes, the ob/gyn who has treated her in the past might not be the best person to handle the pregnancy. Some doctors might do everything but deliveries (not all doctors in ob/gyn practices deliver).

If you have a high-risk pregnancy, then her regular ob/gyn might not be the best fit—you may need a specialist. A doctor who prefers medically-assisted births might not be a good fit for someone who wants a nonmedicated natural birth. Likewise, a woman who wants a medically-assisted birth might not want a doctor who encourages a more holistic approach. There are also issues like the size of the practice, location of the practice, where she wants to deliver (hospital, birthing center, home), and if insurance offers you the freedom to pick and choose your doctor (some doctors might be out of network, and therefore much more expensive).

When it comes to the number of doctors in the practice, size can matter. Some women find large practices less personal and are uncomfortable with not knowing who will show up on the day she goes into labor. Some may find a smaller practice lacking in resources and support services. There are pros and cons associated with both. As for who will deliver the baby, ask your doctor about the percentage of time he or she actually is present for the big day and decide if those odds work for you.

NOTE: My wife's doctor didn't deliver the baby, but the other doctor who did the delivery was awesome. We thought that knowing in advance who would deliver the baby was a big deal, but turned out not to be a big deal—shocking, I know. We literally met the delivering doctor an hour before our daughter was born and loved our experience.

Again, you should be able to ask questions and get answers without feeling like you're being annoying (to speak up if you feel uncomfortable). When choosing the doctor, she should be completely comfortable, and make sure that you're comfortable. Discuss your birth plan (see Tip #73) and make sure the doctor's style and bedside manner are in alignment with both of your needs.

THE MIDWIFE

A midwife isn't a doctor or a wife (although she can be married). There are two kinds of midwives in the United States: certified nurse-midwives and direct-entry midwives. According to the American College of Nurse-Midwives (ACNM), "Certified nurse-midwives are registered nurses who have graduated from a nurse-midwifery education program accredited by the

ACNM Division of Accreditation (DOA) and have passed a national certification examination to receive the professional designation of certified nurse-midwife." A direct-entry midwife does not have the nursing training and cannot prescribe medication. A direct-entry midwife can also be called a certified professional midwife (if certified with the North American Registry of Midwives [NARM]).

A midwife approaches pregnancy differently than many doctors. The midwife's approach is one of mind and body. A midwife will speak to the needs of the expectant mother (and father) on a personal, spiritual, and medical level. She wants you and your partner to be completely at ease and connected with the care and process.

Some doctors work with midwives. If you're worried about a midwife taking over your role as a labor partner, don't be. Most midwives will encourage you to be as large a part of the process as you want to be. A midwife is definitely an option worth exploring.

THE DOULA

The doula is a partner during delivery, a birth coach, an advocate, and a trusted ally. She may work with you and your partner extensively prior to delivery, or just meet with you briefly and show up when your partner goes into labor. A doula typically focuses on the comfort of the mother by doing things like offering an explanation of what's going on during labor and delivery, offering words of encouragement, rubbing her back during labor, or even holding the mother's hand. Like a midwife, the doula wants partners to be part of the experience.

While a doula doesn't deliver the baby, the doula is there for the delivery with the doctor or midwife. The doula knows the playbook and can offer tips, strategies, and insights that will help execute the birth plan. There is research that points to a reduced rate of C-sections, episiotomies, and complications with doula-assisted births. The doula is focused on creating the most comfortable, healthy, and empowering experience for the mother *and* father. When investigating a doula, visit DONA International at www.doula.org. A doula can cost between $300 to $1,200, depending on her level of involvement.

THE BOTTOM LINE:
The doctor who knows his or her business might not be the right doctor to do the business of labor and delivery. If your partner wants a midwife or doula, don't let the names scare you—they want to support you, not control you.

Tip #5
WHERE TO HAVE IT: Birthing Centers, Hospitals, Homes, Cars, Cabs, Sidewalks…

THE TIP:
Having the birth in a hospital setting is just one option.

THE STORY:

After having two children in a hospital setting, we weighed the risks and we decided to have our third one at home—it was a dramatic difference. As a chiropractor, I've held a very naturalistic philosophy around health and wellness. It is beyond me that we treat the birth process as a medical condition. When I looked at the history of women giving birth, most births did not happen in a hospital. I've always thought of the hospital as a place for someone who is sick. It didn't make sense from my point of view to have another hospital birth. At home, it was far more relaxed, no rushing, and it all happened at a natural time. If a problem came up during the delivery, the doctor would have seen it coming. There was a medical van waiting in the driveway just in case. The birth went off without a hitch.

—Stuart, father of three girls (9, 6, and 2)

You can do it in a hospital, at a birthing center, at home, or some place in between (avoid airplanes, buses, and cabs). We knew we would have our baby in the hospital before the urine hit the pregnancy test strip. Everyone we know who has given birth has done it in a hospital—friends, family, parents, etc. I just assumed that everyone did it in a hospital. It wasn't until writing this book that I realized there were other options.

I'm still a hospital birth kind of guy. As a first-time dad, the care and attention of a hospital setting was comforting. That said, a hospital is a medical center—no question about it. There are nurses checking in, staff attending to the room, and doctors coming and going. Then there are visiting hours, a checkout time, and other rules and regulations. And it can be a challenge for caregivers to deviate from their usual routine to accommodate your birth plan. As helpful as we found the attention and constant care, other people I spoke with found it intrusive.

Considering that a hospital birth is the most common place to deliver, the idea of *not* giving birth at a hospital might freak you out (or your family). If your pregnant partner wants to explore something other than a hospital birth, don't freak out. (Your family physician may also be qualified to perform deliveries. Home births will often be facilitated by a family physician.) Do some research and get a better handle on it. For low-risk births, there can be healthy alternatives. Whatever you decide, talk to people who have done it before, who have a similar sensibility, and have followed a similar birth plan. The birth plan includes things like whether or not she wants an epidural, who you want present in the labor and delivery room, and postpartum care. Once you know what you want, you can let that guide you to the right venue to have the baby (see Tip #73 for information on birth plans). For information about birthing centers, you can check out www.birthcenter.org.

BIRTHING CENTERS

A birthing center is the closest thing to home without being at home. Birthing centers can be attached to a hospital, next to a hospital, or freestanding. They are typically for women interested in having natural births who have a low risk of complications. Care is most frequently provided by a certified nurse-midwife, a direct-entry midwife, or a nurse. Birth centers do not perform any "routine" medical procedures. A fetal monitor and IV are not necessarily part of a birthing center birth, but they can be available. By doing away with most high-tech equipment and routine procedures, labor and birth remain a natural and personal process. If you are interested in delivering at a birthing center, make sure it is accredited by the Commission for the Accreditation of Birth Centers. Accredited birthing centers must have affiliated doctors at a nearby hospital in case problems arise with the mom or baby.

QUESTIONS YOU SHOULD ASK

- Does the hospital offer birthing classes? How many? Cost?
- What kind of paperwork needs to be completed?
- Will my medical information be here? Do we need to bring a copy?

- Are there birth balls, music players, or other amenities?
- What types of medication are available?
- What is the procedure for administering anesthesia? Are epidurals available?
- Is anesthesia available 24 hours?
- Is there a neonatal intensive care unit on site?
- Does the hospital encourage natural labor or induced labor (using Pitocin)?
- How is labor monitored (type of fetal monitoring devices)?
- Is this a teaching hospital with residents?
- What are the rates of induction, episiotomy, epidurals, C-sections, and forceps-assisted and vacuum-assisted births?
- Are doulas available?
- Who ensures the birth plan is followed? Procedures?
- Can we take photos and/or videos during the birth?

COMFORT IS SUBJECTIVE:

If your partner wants a medical team down the hall "just in case," a hospital birth can be comfortable. If your partner wants a medical team down the street "just in case," another location can be comfortable.

- What are the visiting hours and rules regarding number of visitors at one time?
- What are the C-section procedures? Can dad be there? Doula? Is baby given to mom immediately?
- Following labor, is the room private?
- Can people stay overnight? Average length of stay (usually longer after C-section)?
- Is a lactation consultant available?
- Does baby stay in mom's room or in the nursery?

THE BOTTOM LINE:
The right place to give birth is where you and your partner can be comfortable, calm, and cared for—and covered by insurance (a nice bonus).

Tip #6
HOW TO PAY FOR IT: Now Is a Good Time to Check Your Insurance

THE TIP:
Discuss coverage for the baby with a health insurance agent. Saving a few hundred dollars today could cost you tomorrow.

THE STORY:
My wife was working full time before she got pregnant. She had much better health benefits than I did. She was planning on quitting once she had the baby.

We were all set to put the baby on her policy because it was hundreds of dollars cheaper and a better all-around policy. Our insurance agent advised us not to be so quick to put the baby under her coverage. If he was on my wife's policy and she quit her job, then both she and the baby would need insurance. If the baby had some sort of birth defect, getting insurance could be hard. Having a baby with special needs makes it complicated. Putting him under my policy meant that no matter what, he would be covered without excluding preexisting conditions.

—Danny, son 21 months

✳ ✳ ✳

WARNING:
If changing coverage, inquire about waiting periods. Some health insurance providers have waiting periods before maternity coverage kicks in. You might have to wait twelve months until maternity coverage takes effect, which means you're effectively on your own if birth control fails.

If you want to make this health insurance section more fun, play some music in the background, drink a beer, or read it during a sporting event (although if you're attending the event with your friends and you read about health insurance they might get pissed, especially if someone is taking you to the game).

Assuming you're reading this after finding out the news that you're expecting, it's not going to help much to tell you that maternity care isn't always part of insurance coverage. (Wow, I think I just heard someone scream.) If you find out that your partner is not covered, there's some good news. A lot of hospitals, labs, and healthcare providers will offer substantial discounts to individuals paying out of pocket. Assistance might also be available through the state or federal government (depending on your level of income). Should you ever get a bill, ask the provider for a discount. When we were charged a lot for genetic testing (see Tip #12), the lab took off 30 percent just because I asked. All you have to do is ask, and they'll typically give you a break on most medical bills (not just genetic testing).

Assuming you have coverage, reacquaint yourself with your policy's rules and regulations. If you have a health insurance agent, give him or her a call. If you want to call the insurance provider directly, that works too. You're going to want to find out what your coverage includes so you can make the right moves. Some insurance companies require that you notify them immediately after finding out that you're expecting. Some want to know when you check into the hospital for delivery. Others have rules that must be followed to ensure coverage (or you could end up with penalties and bills).

When it comes to issues like method of delivery, type of care, and location of care provided, make sure you know what will be covered. It's a bad idea to begin investigating these questions after the baby is born or while passing time during labor because...well, because that's just not responsible (although never investigating would be even less responsible). Find out things like the number of ultrasounds covered by your plan, whether your hospital is in network, and what kind of prenatal care is provided as soon as possible. Contact your healthcare provider or health insurance agent and make sure you're covered. When dealing with insurance providers, ask to get information in writing (email works). In addition, make sure you get the name of the person you speak with and their identification number. Keep a notebook and title it "Important Conversations" (or whatever you want to call it). Should you end up in a disagreement with your insurance provider, having names and ID numbers will prove invaluable.

QUESTIONS YOU SHOULD ASK
- What does your health care coverage include?
- What kind of prenatal tests are covered (and how many ultrasounds)?
- Is preauthorization required for any prenatal or maternal care?
- What is your deductible (the amount you will be responsible for paying before the insurance company begins to pay the bills)?

- What percentage of the bill will you have to pay? (You might have to pay a percentage of the cost based on the type of plan you have. Twenty percent can be a lot to budget for.)
- Is the doctor or midwife part of the plan? (Not all doctors are in network.)
- Do they cover midwives, doulas, or other services?
- Does coverage include birthing centers and home births?
- Do you need to contact your health insurance provider when admitted into the hospital?
- If you need a longer stay due to medical issues, what is the procedure?
- Does your coverage include a private room or semi-private room? Cost to upgrade?
- What hospitals are in network and out of network? (In-network hospitals have agreements with the insurance provider; out-of-network hospitals are not always covered as thoroughly and can be more complicated.)
- Do they cover cord blood storage or offer a discount?
- What is the procedure to add coverage for the newborn? (Generally this has to be done within thirty days of the birth.)
- What does the coverage include once the baby is born?
- What are the rules regarding a pediatrician who is either in or out of network?

- Is lactation counseling covered?
- Does coverage include circumcision? What about once the baby leaves the hospital?

QUESTIONS TO DISCUSS WITH YOUR PARTNER:

- Will the baby be on your policy or her policy? (If she's going to stop working and you're on her policy, make sure you have coverage and that the baby has coverage. Set it up *now*.)
- Do you have a pediatrician in mind? Is he or she in your network?
- What vaccines do you want the baby to receive?
- Do you want to do cord blood storage? (See Tip #77)

LOST YOUR COVERAGE?

If you lose your job, change jobs, or lose coverage during pregnancy, investigate COBRA (Consolidated Omnibus Budget Reconciliation Act) insurance. COBRA gives workers and their families who lose their health benefits the right to choose to continue group health benefits provided by their group health plan for limited periods of time under certain circumstances such as voluntary or involuntary job loss, reduction in the hours worked, transition between jobs, death, divorce, and other life events. Qualified individuals may be required to pay the entire premium

LOST YOUR COVERAGE? (Contd.)

for coverage up to 102 percent of the cost of the plan. COBRA generally requires that group health plans sponsored by employers with twenty or more employees in the prior year offer employees and their families the opportunity for a temporary extension of health coverage (called continuation coverage) in certain instances where coverage under the plan would otherwise end. It could cost a little more, but it's a short-term solution that can save you in the long run.

(Source: http://www.dol.gov/dol/topic/health-plans/cobra.htm)

KEY INSURANCE TERMS

HMO: Stands for Health Maintenance Organization. An HMO consists of an organization of healthcare providers (doctors and hospitals) that offer their services at a fixed price and are contracted with an insurance company. The rules and restrictions of HMO plans can be limiting. Your primary care physician will manage your health care and must be a member of the HMO. This means you might need a new doctor in the network (if your current doctor isn't in network). In order to see a specialist, your primary care physician must be the one to refer you, but you can always go out of network and pay additional fees.

PPO: Stands for Preferred Provider Organization. A PPO consists of a more loosely organized group of doctors and hospitals that have a contractual relationship with an insurance company. A PPO gives you the flexibility to see whichever doctor you choose. You have the option to select an out-of-network physician, but you will have to pay more out of pocket. You also don't need a referral to see a specialist. PPOs cost more than HMOs, but many people choose them because they are far less restrictive.

IN-NETWORK PROVIDER: A care provider who has an agreement with the insurance provider.

OUT-OF-NETWORK PROVIDER: A care provider who doesn't have an agreement with the insurance provider.

PREMIUM: The amount you pay for coverage.

DEDUCTIBLE: The amount you have to pay before the insurance company picks up the bill.

MEDICAID: Government-subsidized coverage for low-income families.

COST OF CARE
According to a study released by the March of Dimes Foundation (2004 data):

- Average expenditures for maternity care were $7,737 for vaginal delivery, of which about $7,205 was paid by private health plans and $463 in out-of-pocket costs was paid by the family.
- Average expenditures for maternity care were $10,958 for C-section delivery, of which about $10,324 was paid by private health plans and $523 in out-of-pocket costs was paid by the family.

- Vaginal delivery costs were distributed in the following way: 48% facility fees, 36% professional service fees, 8% radiology and imaging, 5% outpatient drug, and 4% laboratory.
- C-section delivery costs were distributed in the following way: 53% facility fees, 32% professional service fees, 7% radiology and imaging, 4% outpatient drug, and 3% laboratory.
- It is most expensive to have a baby in the Northeast, least expensive in the South, and the same pattern holds for C-section and vaginal deliveries. Average expenditures for vaginal delivery by geographical region were: $8,718 in the Northeast; $7,455 in the South; $7,501 in the North Central region; and $7,880 in the West. Average expenditures for C-section delivery were: $12,175 in the Northeast; $10,317 in the South; $10,969 in the North Central region; and $11,581 in the West.

LIFE OR DISABILITY INSURANCE

Chances are you will live a full life. But there's always the most remote chance that you might get hit by a bus (while checking your email on your phone to see if she's in labor yet). If you do meet a bus, or some unpredictable and highly unlikely demise, it's comforting to think that you will still be able to provide for your family. Life insurance and disability insurance are *not* about you. It's about the people who rely on you financially and emotionally. The last thing anyone needs during a stressful emotional time is a stressful financial emotional time. And that's what insurance is for. Some people don't want to get life or disability insurance because it implies death or tragedy and some people hate the idea of death or tragedy, but it's about enabling those you love to maintain their lifestyle.

The general rule is that you want enough insurance to enable your family to maintain their lifestyle and take care of financial obligations (mortgage, child care, loans, car payments). How much insurance you'll need to get varies, but get it. Talk to a qualified agent or financial planner to discuss your individual needs. You might be thinking that the last thing you can afford is life insurance, but once you check it out, you'll be surprised at how inexpensive it can be. Assuming you're in relatively good health, we're talking less than a monthly telephone bill. And while you're talking

PREGNANCY Q & A:

QUESTION: Any medical surprises? ANSWER: The doctor mentioned my uterus was a little big and I could be having twins. We don't know yet. We are waiting for the first ultrasound and since our insurance only covers one, we want to have it later so that we can find out the sex at the same time. My husband is very excited and hopes for twins. I hope he won't be disappointed. (Tiffany, 7 weeks pregnant) about life insurance, look into disability insurance. While you never want to use insurance, it's comforting to know that if something should happen, you'll be assured that your family will be taken care of.

THE BOTTOM LINE:
If your doctor requires cash, check to see if there's an ATM in the delivery room. If you find an ATM in the delivery room, you're probably in an ATM lobby and should get to the nearest hospital.

Tip #7
FEEDING YOUR PREGNANT PARTNER: Keep your fingers far away from her mouth…

THE TIP:
Don't question cravings—just get her what she wants. There's no talking through cravings. None of it is rational.

THE STORY:
I got constant food cravings. The cravings can be weird. With my first, I couldn't get enough orange juice. With the second, it's been chocolate. There's no rational reason—it just happens. Not only did I get cravings, but food aversions. During the first trimester, I was sick or nauseous and I couldn't stomach eating meat. I couldn't prepare it. I couldn't be around it. I

couldn't look at it. Chicken was the worst. The sight of all meat absolutely repulsed me. I'm telling you, raw meat was disgusting, gross, nasty, and horrible. I ate peanut butter and jelly and grilled cheese sandwiches for weeks. My husband didn't ask me to explain, and that's a good thing, because I couldn't explain it. He just went with the flow. Once I hit 25 weeks, it all started to go away. A few weeks later, I was in full force eating steak, chicken, and all those things I loved. It's not logical or rational—gosh no, but it's just how it was.

—Denise, daughter 21 months, 32 weeks pregnant

✳ ✳ ✳

If you're reading this part of the book while feeding your pregnant partner a chunk of blue cheese, raw tuna, undercooked bacon, cookie batter (with raw egg), and a glass of warm, fresh squeezed cow's milk (unpasteurized) moments after cleaning the kitty litter box with your bare hands (the hands you're now feeding your partner with), throw down this book and scream for her to stop eating! Wash your hands with soap and warm water immediately (scrub for at least thirty seconds).

Welcome back.

Don't try to understand—just go with it. Last pregnancy she wanted orange soda and gyros every day for a month, and she *hates* gyros. Won't even look at them now. This time it's orange sherbet and grilled cheese sandwiches with sweet pickles. Gotta be gherkins.
—Patrick (expecting baby #6)

A lot of expectant fathers will find that pregnant women get ravenously hungry. When the hunger hits, they need to be satisfied. (Keep food next to the bed or in the bed if it's a big enough bed to avoid a 3:00 a.m. wake-up call and run to the kitchen.) The problem is that your pregnant partner might not be able to feed herself. Sometimes you'll have to be the one to cook, order, or shop for the food. Some men are already great cooks, but a lot aren't. If you're used to having her cook for you, this could be a tough transition.

I contemplated including menus in this section of the book to help you prepare some basic meals for her, but I know that I'd never use menus from an expectant father book. More importantly, a pregnant woman's palate changes minute by minute. So, if you want to cook, ask her what she wants and search online for a recipe. You'll get easy recipes that need very few ingredients. If she doesn't eat it, don't be offended. She might see it or smell it and realize she can't bear to eat it (don't take it personally if she vomits).

Of course, the easiest way to feed her is to order it. If you do order in, make sure you know what you should and shouldn't feed her. This might mean asking the people on the phone lots of questions. (If you don't like being annoying, do your own cooking because asking for special orders on the phone can mean being annoying at times.) When ordering, it helps to tell them she's pregnant. You're not the first guy calling in a pregnant order. Then again, you might have someone new and clueless on the phone. I don't mind asking people questions about whether cheese is pasteurized, if raw eggs are in the Caesar salad dressing, or if they can prepare the cooked sushi far away from the raw fish (on a separate board with separate cutlery) and package the cooked rolls away from the raw ones.

As for her cravings, they might not be so irrational. Pregnant women require more folic acid, iron, calcium, and water. While a prenatal vitamin should take care of the essentials (make sure she's taking prenatal vitamins), certain foods might be calling her name because the baby is craving essential nutrients. Orange juice, leafy greens, and dried beans are all rich in folic acid. That steak is rich in iron. That ice cream is rich in calcium—it might take a pint a day of Ben & Jerry's for her to get enough of it (and yes, there are better choices).

PREGNANCY TRIVIA:

CATEGORY: Extra Calories Pregnant Women Need

QUESTION: How many additional calories does a pregnant woman need to consume on a daily basis?
a) 300 calories,
b) 600 calories,
c) 1,800 calories,
d) 3,600 calories (For the answer, see The Bottom Line.)

CAFFEINE:

When surprising her with a latte, make sure it's a decaf. Some studies show that drinking caffeine during pregnancy can harm the fetus. Other research suggests that small amounts of caffeine are safe. Talk to your doctor before encouraging her to drink caffeinated beverages during pregnancy. Caffeine can be found in many over-the-counter and prescription drugs.

Appreciate that a pregnant woman *cannot* eat everything she used to eat before getting pregnant. She might not be able to eat everything you want her to eat (that's why they make prenatal vitamins). Some problem foods include: undercooked meats, deli meats (unless heated to the point where they're steaming), unpasteurized cheese (never blue cheese), and certain seafood (unless it's been cooked, *not* only cured). When preparing fruits and vegetables, make sure they're washed extremely well. Also, keep cutlery, cutting boards, spatulas, plates, and dishes used to prepare raw foods far away from cooked foods (to prevent cross contamination). If you're unsure how long a food has been in the fridge or if it's been sitting out too long, apply the "when in doubt, throw it out" rule.

For a list of questionable foods, visit: http://www.cfsan.fda.gov/~pregnant/pregnant.html. For a list of good foods, visit: http://www.4women.gov/pregnancy/pregnancy/eat.cfm. Need an easy recipe? Google "Easy (fill in the blank with the food item she craves)." When it comes to food-borne illness, the big three concerns are: Listeria, methylmercury, and Toxoplasma gondii (see the FDA website for full definitions). According to the CDC, pregnant women are about 20 times more likely to get listeriosis than other healthy adults and 85 percent of pregnant women in the U.S. are at risk of being infected with toxoplasmosis (do not let her handle that cat litter).

THE BOTTOM LINE:

If she craves it, and it's not dangerous for her to eat it, then find it, cook it, or order it.

MEDICATIONS:

If she gets sick during the pregnancy and she wants you to give her medication, check with your caregiver first. Something like herbal tea seems harmless, but some teas are better than others. She should always talk with her doctor before taking any drugs or medicines while pregnant. If you look online for help, make sure it's a trusted and reputable source. Normal medications she took before getting pregnant can pose a risk now.

Don't ask her questions about it. Especially not a trivia question about the number of additional calories she should be consuming—and the answer to the trivia question is: a) She needs 300 additional calories a day.

Tip #8
THE PREGNANCY CARD: Use It, Don't Abuse It

(**NOTE:** read this tip to your pregnant partner)

THE TIP:
Being pregnant isn't a ticket to do whatever you want for nine months.

THE STORY:
I've witnessed it personally. It happens—usually with a woman who is high-maintenance to begin with. I have friends who joke about using their pregnancy to get their husbands to do things because they can. They'll talk about not wanting to do something and having their husbands clean, or cook, or do something because they just don't feel like doing it. I remember receiving a card when I got pregnant that said, "Congratulations, now you have an excuse to never lift a finger for nine months." Personally, I never flashed my pregnancy card—at least I don't think I have. I asked my husband to do things out of need, not because I was taking advantage of being pregnant. There were plenty of times I needed help. Eventually, a guy will just say forget it. It's a balancing act—I'm not one to abuse it.

—Anne, daughter 1 year, son 3½ years

✳ ✳ ✳

Now that she's pregnant, she's going to expect certain things. Newly pregnant women can become consumed with their newfound power and will use, and sometimes abuse, The Pregnancy Card. This is the card a pregnant woman can pull at any time, anywhere, and for whatever reason she sees fit. How it works: The other night, as she was getting ready to go to sleep, my wife asked me to get her cell phone charger from the kitchen. I was in bed, about to drift off. I didn't move and she asked me again...only this time she pulled out The Pregnancy Card. She said, "Can you get my charger? I'm really tired and *pregnant*." That's The Pregnancy Card. When it's pulled, a man must move fast and not ask questions. If you do ask questions, you'll get yelled at or look insensitive.

As the author of a book about being an expectant father, I jumped out of bed and asked her a question. I wanted to know if she was really too tired to go downstairs or just pulling a Pregnancy Card. She admitted she was tired, but she shouldn't have used The Pregnancy Card. At 7 weeks, she knew better than to pull the card for something I would have done without her flashing it. She could have gotten what she wanted simply by flashing The Tired Wife Card.

And that brings me to the main reason why I suggested reading this tip with your partner—some pregnant women have been known to abuse The Pregnancy Card. Abuse is when a pregnant woman can do something for herself, but uses her pregnancy to force her partner to action. Asking you to do something isn't the problem. It's reminding you that she's pregnant when asking you. The problem with abusing The Pregnancy Card is that when she really does need something, the card may become ineffective.

It's natural to test the power of the card early on, but absolute power can absolutely go to some pregnant women's heads. I know some pregnant women might think a man should do whatever she demands, but there is such a thing as abuse. It's the same as abusing food—a woman who uses her pregnancy as a license to eat everything and anything on the planet is a pregnant woman who will end up gaining a crazy amount of weight. A pregnant woman who uses her pregnancy to boss around her partner is a pregnant woman who might wear her man down and have him build up resentment. Once that baby is born, you're going to *need* him—pace yourself.

We can never know what it feels like to be pregnant, but pregnant women work, drive, work out, tend the fields, drive buses, wait tables, cook, and function on a high level. Sure, there are times when doing basic functions will be harder than others, and we're always here to help. But that's why it's so important to never abuse The Pregnancy Card.

THE BOTTOM LINE:

Dear Pregnant Women of the World,

We love you and adore you. We are grateful for you and everything you do for us. We are in awe of your magnificence. One request: please act responsibly when flashing The Pregnancy Card. Use us—but please do not abuse us.

Sincerely,
Expectant Fathers of the World

2

THE DOCTOR WILL SEE YOU NOW

Or Whoever Delivers Your Baby Will See You Now

Tip #9
YOUR FIRST GUYNE EXAM: Shake Hands with the Doctor (Then Wash)

THE TIP:
Shock and awe are the best words to describe the first doctor's visit.

THE STORY:
Going to the first visit with my wife wasn't optional. It was expected that I would be in the examination room. I was sitting near the doctor and had a good view of everything. I was expecting the jelly on the

belly like you see in TV. First the doctor inserted a shiny object and checked things out. Then the doctor lubed up a huge probe and shoved it inside her—well, gently placed it inside her. This was the shocking part. My wife made a face but didn't seem to be in pain. Then we saw the images on the screen and a fluttering object. The doctor did more exploring and pointed out that the fluttering was the heart beating. This was the awe part.

—*Scot, daughter 14 months*

* * *

Once the ten pregnancy tests reveal positive results, your partner will make a doctor's appointment. Some doctors will have her come in right away; others will have her wait until week 7 or so to check in. The first exam typically includes the weight check, urine sample, blood pressure, blood work, medical history, and often, a vaginal ultrasound.

What's different about this appointment is that not only will you be invited to attend, you will get a front row seat in the examination room. A seat so close you might see her cervix, or something close to it. (**NOTE:** If you were planning to snap photos, this is not the appointment to bring the camera equipment.) Walking into the gynecologist's waiting room is like walking into a women's bathroom by mistake—when you arrive, a part of you will want to turn around. But you're supposed to be here. It will get easier. The first time is the hardest.

After waiting in the waiting room (an appropriate name for it), you'll be invited into the exam room. You'll see stirrups, instruments (the metal bird beak), lubrication, and a box of condomlike things. As you settle into your seat, your partner will get her blood pressure checked and she will be weighed. She might ask you to leave the room during her weight check. Before the doctor arrives, she will likely be instructed to get naked from the waist down. You should stay clothed. When she starts to get undressed, you'll notice that watching her is about as romantic as watching a grandparent get naked. It's as if her naked body has been transformed, especially her vagina. It won't give off that familiar vagina vibe you know and love. It will look different. It will change. What you're seeing is the birthing vagina (BV). The BV is different than the SV (sex vagina). Not being turned on by the sight of the BV might be distressing at first, but you will learn to separate the BV from the SV over time (more about the split personality of the vagina later). I should mention, some guys might like both the BV and SV—but the first time a man sees the BV can be distressing.

When the doctor arrives, one of two things will occur: The doctor will welcome you and acknowledge your presence, or the doctor will ignore you as if you're invisible. The latter can be comforting and disturbing— comforting because we don't want to be noticed, disturbing because we deserve to be acknowledged. If the doctor ignores you, there's nothing wrong with introducing yourself to him or her. Considering you're part of the process, the doctor should want to know you. Better to do it sooner rather than in the middle of the exam (shaking hands would be awkward) or when the baby is being delivered (that might be a little too late.)

Once the initial chitchat concludes, the exam will begin. Your pregnant partner is now like a car up on the blocks (stirrups); the doctor will sit down and check out the mechanics. If you find this image disturbing to read about, it might be more disturbing to see (but doesn't have to be). The doctor will insert a duck-billed object called a speculum (a plastic or metal object used to examine the vagina, cervix, and uterus). Depending on your seat, you might see a whole new side of your partner (really, it's not so bad).

If the doctor performs a vaginal ultrasound, you'll see a long probe covered with a condom wave around. (The waving part is something I just made up for effect.) The doctor will lubricate the probe and insert it in her. While you're gasping for air and thinking "What the hell is happening? Wow that's *really* big!", she and the doctor will continue chatting it up. She might grimace a bit as the probe enters, but she'll just keep talking away.

Once the probe is in place, you'll get a glimpse inside her uterus on the video monitor (although you'll probably have no idea what is what). The vaginal ultrasound is performed to see if there is a beating heart—or two, three, four, or five beating hearts (dear God, five?). Once a beating heart has been confirmed, your doctor will leave the room, and your partner will clean up and get dressed.

Afterward you'll have a short talk with the doctor and go over some important information. You'll discuss prenatal issues, talk about foods and activities to avoid (no smoking or alcohol), address your questions, and reveal the due date. (More on this in a sec.) If you have questions for the doctor, ask them. You should be able to talk to this doctor about anything and everything on your mind. If you can't ask questions, that's a problem. You and the doctor are two of the only people who have seen your partner naked from the waist down—and that's a bond that can't be broken (until she delivers and there is a roomful of people seeing all of her). You should be able to talk to the doctor.

At some point during the first guy-necologic appointment, you'll find out the magical due date. Don't be so quick to clear your calendar. This due date is 95 percent wrong. That's right, it's usually totally inaccurate. If you're looking for a guaranteed date, call FedEx (but I would not suggesting having FedEx deliver your baby). The due date is a rough estimate that's calculated by counting 40 weeks from the first day of her last period. The due date can change based on the development of the baby.

DAD DEFINITIONS:

BIRTHING VAGINA (BV): Term for the vagina seen during the birthing process

SEX VAGINA (SV): Term for the vagina seen during your honeymoon

WISDOM FROM PATRICK (SIX-TIME EXPECTANT FATHER, 25+ DOCTOR'S VISITS)

Try not to do anything to aggravate or upset your wife. Don't act like a know-it-all—no matter how many pregnancies you've experienced, every time is a new experience. Always be supportive and compassionate—this means doing a whole lot of listening rather than talking. Make sure she knows that what she's saying is important to you. Undivided attention is a key component that is sometimes forgotten due to nervousness. The visual aspect is definitely intimidating. I would compare it to staring directly into the sun. You don't want your eyeballs to catch on fire, but man, isn't sunshine a great thing? No pelvic exams for me. It's uncomfortable enough for her, I would imagine, and privacy far outweighs her need for my presence. (My wife agrees.) Be a friend, hold her hand, and try to be sensitive. Her needs should be more important than your own at this time. I've learned this the hard way. I have made many mistakes; the worst one was being preoccupied with my own feelings and not being very supportive of hers. Pregnancy is stressful enough without hurting her feelings.

THE BOTTOM LINE:

The birthing vagina (BV) is different than the sex vagina (SV). It takes forty weeks and a delivery to complete the transformation. Following the delivery, it takes another eight weeks for the transformation from BV to SV to be completed.

If the due date is only right 5 percent of the time, why not change it to the due week? Or make it a due month? Or just throw a dart at the calendar month the baby is due. While we have touch screen technology, GPS tracking, and video games that make us jump around like morons in our living rooms, we still can't figure out when a baby will be born. Yes, humbling.

THE TIP:

If your partner asks you to come to the prenatal appointments, make an effort to be at the prenatal appointments.

THE STORY:

When I asked him to come with me to the appointments, he wasn't open to the idea. He told me that the prenatal appointments weren't that important for him to go to because all the ob/gyn does is measure my belly and check the heartbeat. His reaction was maddening because in my eyes he should be there. It's his baby too. Being there would have helped him gain a better understanding of what I'm going through. All my hormonal changes become very trying for both of us and having him there would have helped. I wish he would have known how much it meant to me.

—Jessica, 21 weeks pregnant

* * *

Some guys go to all of the appointments. Some guys don't go to all of them. Some guys want to go to all of them but can't go to any of them. I'd say go to as many as you can. Ask your partner what she wants. Make sure you have an idea of when the most important ones will take place.

After the first appointment, she will likely see the doctor once a month during the first six months of pregnancy. Then it's every two weeks in the seventh and eighth months. Then it's every week during the ninth month. If you have all the time and flexibility to go, it's worth going to every appointment. Going to the doctor's visits aren't just about being there for her, it's a way for you to stay connected and keep up. It's like going to class. Hearing about it and getting the notes isn't the same (and your grade will suffer).

The big ones include the first appointment (when you get to see the heartbeat) and the 20-week ultrasound. If your doctor does the nuchal translucency screening (NTS) test, which assesses your baby's risk for Down syndrome and some other medical conditions, there will be an ultrasound around weeks

Whenever I asked questions, I felt like the doctor was thinking, "Why are you speaking?" I just wanted to understand what was happening. When we went to the vet to have our Chihuahua's teeth cleaned, he talked to us for an hour about the two types of anesthesia they use to attack part of the nervous subsystem. The vet gave us ten thousand times more information than we got from the doctor delivering our child. We were thinking of having the vet deliver the next one.
—Anthony (daughter 3 weeks)

Our doctor made it extremely easy to ask questions. He always asked me if there was anything on my mind. I think he was asking for my benefit, but also so he could get a sense of how my wife was feeling through my eyes.
—Andy (son 21 months)

11–13. The other big ones include whichever ones she wants you to attend. (Attending the birth is also a good idea.) There might not be an obvious reason for you to go (in your eyes), but just being there helps her feel supported.

The doctor will check the progress of the baby. He'll measure her belly. He'll put her on the scale (leave the room if she wants). Later on, he'll check her cervix. He'll talk about the tests he's performing. He'll go through her wishes regarding the birth plan (more in Tip #73). He'll answer her questions. And hopefully he'll address your questions.

Sometimes pregnant women can be forgetful; if you're there with her, you can help her remember to ask the questions she may forget. I used to write a list before the appointment as a backup just in case one of us forgot to ask about something. When it comes to the questions part of the appointment, ask your partner if she wants you to leave the room. There might be things she's just not up for mentioning in front of you—like the increased vaginal discharge she's been experiencing.

My boss told me to take as much time as I wanted at doctor's appointments during the pregnancy because it all goes so fast. My wife made appointments in the early morning or late afternoon. This way, I could go before work or leave work early and catch the train.

—*Jeff (son 9 months)*

Things to keep in mind:

- The caregiver who examines her might not be the caregiver who delivers the baby. Ours wasn't.
- Suggest having her schedule the *big* appointments first thing in the morning or last thing in the

afternoon. Weekends are good too.

- Caregivers can be intimidating. If your caregiver is impatient while answering your questions, say something. Most of them don't realize they're doing anything wrong. Let them know if you have a problem.

- If you can't attend an appointment, ask about it. Get her some flowers or a card, or cook dinner to let her know you wish you could have been there. She'll never be happier you didn't go.

THE BOTTOM LINE:

Being there means having a sense of what's happening and what's going to happen. It will make you calmer and send the message that you want to be involved, which will make her more comfortable.

PREGNANCY Q & A:

QUESTION: What percentage of the doctor's appointments did you attend?
ANSWER: For the first one, 100 percent; for the second one, 50 percent; for the third one, I think I went once and that was when the baby was born. (Matt, father of three)

Tip #11

THE TIP:
Make sure to attend the ultrasound appointments and make sure you get a good night's sleep the night before.

THE STORY:
My wife and I have chosen not to find out the baby's gender, so when it got to the point in the sonogram where the technician said she was going to find out the gender and put it in the file, I closed my eyes. The room was dark, there was a dull rumble from the air-conditioning, and I had not gotten much sleep the night before. When I woke up, my wife was staring daggers at me and no amount of apologies or loving statements could assuage her (well-deserved) anger. Man, what an asshole I was! Now I make sure that whenever she says the baby is kicking I run to feel for myself, mostly because I want to feel it kicking but partly because I want her to know I am very much interested in what is happening with our baby.

—Lou, 26 weeks pregnant

He's an EMT. Nothing surprised him, but he did tear up during the ultrasound.

—Nancy (daughter 15 months)

✳ ✳ ✳

The ultrasound is a must-see event—like *Cats* (the musical), but better. It's worth bringing the whole family. It's not quite the World Series, but it's a league championship.

If you can only attend two doctor's visits, make it the first appointment when you find out the news and the 18- to 20-week ultrasound. If your work schedule makes attending appointments rough, have her schedule the ultrasound appointment during the first visit so you have time to plan ahead. If getting time off from work is tough, suggest that she make the appointment first thing in the morning, late in the afternoon, or on the weekend.

How many ultrasounds you have depends on your caregiver, your insurance (check your coverage), and how the pregnancy progresses. The norm tends to be two to three (sometimes only one). A high-risk pregnancy will likely result in a higher number of ultrasounds.

We had three ultrasounds during our typical pregnancy. The first was a vaginal ultrasound (long probe). This ultrasound confirmed the pregnancy and showed us the heartbeat. The second ultrasound was at 11 weeks—this was like the one in the movies. Not that they had a

When we went for the 18- to 20-week ultrasound and saw what looked like a little penis pop up, my fiancé gave me a high five and started to do a little dance, saying, "That's my man." When the little boy turned out to be a little girl, and what we had seen turned out to be the umbilical cord, his dance turned into, "Oh well, girls can still be race car drivers."

—*Jessica (pregnant 21 weeks)*

full crew filming it—what I mean is that the doctor put the gel on her belly and rubbed a little mouselike instrument over it. This ultrasound was used to measure the thickness of the skinfold behind the neck (part of the nuchal fold scan—see Tip #12). The third ultrasound happened at 20 weeks. This was performed to make sure everything was developing properly. The doctor looked at the heart, neural tubes, arms, legs, fingers, head, brain, GI tract, and (turn away if you don't want to see) the sex. You can find ultrasound images online to give you a sense of what you'll see and what the doctor will measure. As for gender, it might be possible to determine whether you're having a boy or girl at the 11- to 13-week ultrasound, but the 18- to 20-week one will reveal the sex with a higher probability of accuracy—assuming the kid exposes him- or herself for the camera.

Up until the first ultrasound, the pregnancy might not seem real. I mean, I knew it was real, but seeing that beating heart at the 7-week exam and hearing the heartbeat at the 11-week ultrasound is *really* real. For me, it marked the beginning of the emotional connection. To see it is to believe it. To believe it is to feel it. At the 11-week ultrasound, we not only saw it, we heard it. At 20 weeks, the baby looks like a little person. We saw it sucking its thumb and rolling around in the uterus.

Record the 20-week ultra-sound if possible. You might not think about bringing a VHS tape or a DVD, but your doctor might have a VHS or DVD recorder hooked up to the ultrasound machine. Call the office before you arrive and see if they have something available to record it. If they don't have a recording device, bring a video camera with you. Once you find out that everything is perfect, you can use your video camera (or camera phone) to record the images of your baby on the screen. Then you can upload it and share it with the family (or not).

THE BOTTOM LINE:

If you can only make it to one appointment, make it to an ultrasound. Plan the date far in advance and coordinate your calendars. If getting time off is not possible, look into a weekend doctor's appointment.

POSSIBLE ULTRASOUND SCHEDULE (SCHEDULE MAY VARY, CONSULT YOUR DOCTOR OR CARE PROVIDER):

7 WEEKS: Confirm pregnancy and count the babies (vaginal ultrasound).

11–13 WEEKS: Nuchal fold scan to identify risks of Down syndrome (and chromosomal abnormalities and major congenital heart problems).

18–20 WEEKS: Time to check for any abnormal development.

Tip #12
PRENATAL TESTING: They Want Her Bodily Fluids, Not Yours (Yet)

THE TIP:
Get tested for genetic disorders. Check with your insurance—sometimes there are programs that can help with the cost.

THE STORY:
Before we got pregnant, my doctor recommended that we do some genetic testing. We are Jewish and therefore have increased odds of being carriers of several genetic disorders like Gaucher's disease, Tay-Sachs disease, cystic fibrosis, and others. I had blood drawn after my annual checkup and was shocked when I was later told that I tested positive for a rare mutation of the Tay-Sachs gene. This meant my husband had to get tested too. If he had tested positive, there was a 25 percent chance the baby could have it and a 50 percent chance the baby would be a carrier. If we both had been carriers, we could still have gotten pregnant, but we would have had to test the baby via amniocentesis or CVS testing. It turned out that he wasn't a carrier, and I'm so grateful we didn't have to go through any of that. The only hassle throughout this whole process was my insurance—arghhhh! They didn't cover the tests at first. It was only after thirty calls and hours of

getting bounced around to different people (I'm not exaggerating) that a helpful rep was able to "suggest" that my doctor code it differently; they then covered the claim! We couldn't get them to cover my husband's test because the insurance said that his tests were experimental. He was able to save a couple hundred dollars by paying in advance and doing it at a hospital that was part of a community-based group for genetic testing.

—Erin, daughter 20 months,
14 weeks pregnant with #2

✳ ✳ ✳

The pregnancy test was just the first test. But that's just the beginning. Some tests are nothing. Others will put your nerves to the test.

If you haven't already had genetic testing before the pregnancy, consider having it done when you find out the news. Genetic testing is a relatively new tool that can help detect the possibility of certain genetic disorders before birth. Three common tests include those for cystic fibrosis, Tay-Sachs disease, and sickle-cell trait. The tests use blood work from the mom to determine if she is a carrier of the disorders. It's ideal to do the testing before getting pregnant, but because pregnancy isn't always something you can predict, your partner can get tested once you get pregnant.

Consult your doctor or a genetic counselor to determine which tests you need. Even if all the tests come back negative, there is still a small chance of being a carrier, although it's extremely unlikely. If any one of the tests comes back positive, the father will then need to get tested for that particular gene. Most genetic disorders need a gene from the mother and the father to be passed along to the baby. And just because both parents are carriers of a given gene doesn't mean the baby will inherit that disorder. The gene may lay dormant or not be passed along. If both parents are carriers of the abnormal cystic fibrosis (CF) gene, there's a 25 percent chance the child will have symptoms of CF, a 50 percent chance the child will be a carrier (and have no symptoms), and a 25 percent chance the child will not be a carrier and not have the disease (see www.cff.org for more information).

Certain ethnic groups and races have higher risks of being carriers. For example, in the United States, sickle-cell anemia affects about 70,000 people. It mainly affects African Americans, with the condition occurring in about 1 out of every 500 African American births. Hispanic Americans also are affected; the condition occurs in 1 out of every 1,000 to 1,400 Hispanic American births. About 2 million Americans have the sickle-cell trait. About 1 in 12 African Americans has the sickle-cell trait. Genetic counseling can help identify risk and guide couples.

The most frustrating aspect about genetic testing is that while it's so valuable, insurance companies can be less than accommodating about covering it. It's hard to understand why genetic testing isn't a routine part of the pregnancy process. While most states screen newborns for cystic fibrosis, sickle-cell anemia, and other genetic disorders at birth, they don't require parents to be screened for the genes that can result in a child being born with these disorders. In a perfect world, genetic testing would be accessible, available, and affordable to everyone. Maybe in the next edition of this book, this story will have a much happier ending.

In addition to genetic testing, there are normal screening tests and various diagnostic tests that may be recommended during the pregnancy. Screening tests determine the risk of having a baby with some genetic birth defects. What's nice about screening tests is that they do not pose any risk to the fetus or mother. But screening tests cannot tell you for sure if the baby has a birth defect. Instead, screening tests tell you the odds of your baby having a birth defect based on your age or other factors (i.e., 1-in-50,000 chance that the child has…).

Diagnostic tests can give definitive "yes" or "no" answers about whether your baby has a particular problem; but unlike screening tests, they are usually invasive or come with a risk of miscarriage. Amniocentesis and chorionic villus sampling (CVS) are the two most commonly used, and both tests are more than 99 percent accurate for determining the presence of these problems; the only negative is that the risk of miscarriage from an amniocentesis or CVS is 1 in 200.

SCREENING TESTS

Some screening and diagnostic tests during pregnancy include (Source: www.4women.gov):

- Targeted ultrasound: The best time to receive this test is between 18 and 20 weeks of pregnancy. Most major problems with the way your baby might be formed can be seen at this time. But some problems like clubbed feet and heart defects can be missed on ultrasound. Your doctor also will be able to see if your baby has any neural tube defects, such as spina bifida. This test is not the most accurate for finding out whether your baby has Down syndrome. Only 1 in 3 babies with Down syndrome have an abnormal second-trimester ultrasound. In most cases, your doctor can find out the sex of your baby through ultrasound.

- Maternal serum marker screening test: This blood test can be called by many different names including multiple marker screening test, triple test, quad screen, and others. This test is usually given between 15 and 20 weeks of pregnancy. It checks for birth defects such as Down syndrome (trisomy 18) or open neural tube defects.

- Nuchal translucency screening (NTS) or nuchal fold scan: This new type of screening can be done between 11 and 14 weeks of pregnancy. It uses an ultrasound and blood test to calculate the risk of some birth defects. Doctors use the ultrasound exam to check the thickness of the back of the fetus's neck. They also test the blood for levels of a pregnancy-associated plasma protein and a hormone called human chorionic gonadotropin (hCG). Doctors use this information to tell if the fetus has a normal or greater-than-normal chance of having some birth defects. (**NOTE:** NTS is not yet widely used. If you are interested in NTS, talk to your doctor. If she is unable to do the test, she can refer you to someone who can. You should also call your insurance company to find out if they cover the cost of this procedure.)

- Glucose screening test: The test is administered around weeks 24–28 to detect gestational diabetes. The patient consumes a drink containing glucose (a form of sugar). If the test shows high blood sugar levels, the woman will need to take a diagnostic test to find out if she has gestational diabetes.

DIAGNOSTIC TESTS

- Amniocentesis: This test is performed in pregnancies of at least 16 weeks. It involves inserting a thin needle through the abdomen, into the uterus, and into the amniotic sac to take out a small amount of amniotic fluid for testing. The cells from the fluid are grown in a lab to look for problems with chromosomes. About 1 in 200 women have a miscarriage as a result of this test.
- Chorionic villus sampling (CVS): This test is performed between weeks 10 and 12 of pregnancy.

HELPFUL GENETIC DISORDER RESOURCES:

National Library of Medicine's Genetic Home Reference site: http://ghr.nlm.nih.gov

Chicago Center for Jewish Genetic Disorders: http://www.jewishgenet-icscenter.org/
(See resources on page 498)

The doctor inserts a needle through the abdomen or inserts a catheter through the cervix in order to reach the placenta. The doctor then takes a sample of cells from the placenta. These cells are sent to a lab to look for problems with the chromosomes. CVS cannot find out whether your baby has open neural tube defects. About 1 in 200 women have a miscarriage as a result of this test.

THE BOTTOM LINE:

Look into genetic testing. If insurance won't cover the testing, contact your local children's hospital and speak to a genetic counselor. There may be testing programs available in the community or a way to code the test so that your health insurance will provide coverage. Just know that testing is an option.

THE TIP:

If there are any questions, GET A SECOND OPINION. What could be more important? If you have access to more brains, use them!

THE STORY:

My wife was on meds from about 20 weeks or so—that's when we found out she had an incompetent cervix. The original doctor we were with wanted to put her on bed rest from that point on, so we went for a second opinion. This guy was a specialist and awesome. He juggled drugs and also put in a support instrument. My wife was being monitored from home for about three months. She wore a monitor, like the one they put on her at the hospital to watch the contractions, twice a day for thirty minutes each time. It counted the contractions, and then transmitted them over the phone to a monitoring agency. If she had more than a certain number of contractions they made her do it again. If she still had more than a certain number of contractions, they called the doctor. It was a major pain, but *way* better than her being stuck on bed rest for the entire three months. In the end, our son came three days before the "due date"—they think he was actually a few days late. I'm just so happy we got a second opinion.

—Adam, son 8 months

* * *

Complications can happen. Some are manageable; others can cause serious risks to the baby and the mother. Later in this chapter, I've included a list of some of the more common complications with short definitions to give you a heads-up. (Check out the *Mayo Clinic Guide to a Healthy Pregnancy* book for more in-depth medical information.)

Should a complication arise, tests may be needed to make or confirm a diagnosis. Some of these tests can put the pregnancy or your partner at risk. Take amniocentesis or CVS testing—both of these tests can be effective in detecting problems such as Down syndrome, spina bifida, and other complications. But the tests have approximately a 1-in-200 risk of resulting in miscarriage. Whether or not to do it, how quickly you need to do it, and who should do it are questions to consider. It

I wish we had known that we don't have to "obey" the doctor. We are having our child and ultimately have to live with the consequences of our decisions. We should have asked what the risks were for different things that the doctor "decided" we needed to do. We should have spoken up and made more informed decisions.

—Lesha (sons 7 months and 3½ years)

might be worth having a caregiver who specializes in a particular procedure perform the test.

Another issue that can come up is bed rest. Factors like having preeclampsia, carrying multiples, or having an incompetent cervix are a few risks that can result in preterm labor. One way to reduce the risk of preterm labor is to be put on bed rest. It can be for days, weeks, or months. Some bed rest can be completely restrictive (only get out of bed to shower and pee). No matter what kind of bed rest, with her in bed, you'll have to be the one in charge of making sure everything is ready for baby.

The tip and story in this section illustrate why it's important to get a second opinion. If your caregiver offers a suggestion that will dramatically impact the pregnancy or your partner's health, consider getting a second opinion. I know this might seem simple, but pregnancy is so emotional, and a lot of women have long relationships with their caregivers. Therefore, suggesting a second opinion might be too sensitive. It's as if you don't trust your caregiver. When facing the unknown, it's comforting to have someone you can trust. And trusting someone means not questioning his or her judgment and creating a possible conflict. On top of this, some caregivers have strong personalities and will make you feel crazy for questioning them. Whereas in other medical situations, we get a second opinion when making difficult medical decisions, during pregnancy it's not always as easy for us to do.

But your comfort level and your partner's comfort level are more important than your caregiver's ego. You and your partner need to be completely sure that what you're doing is the right thing. If a pregnancy becomes complicated, there's *nothing* wrong with consulting a caregiver who has managed similar pregnancies. Some caregivers are more familiar with certain complications and conditions. If your caregiver feels threatened, he's not someone who is being loyal to you.

As the nonchildbearing partner, suggesting a second opinion might not be well received. If you haven't been to many doctor's appointments, it might be less welcome. From her perspective, the last thing she needs is you questioning her doctor's opinion—the doctor she trusts because she's been seeing her since she was sixteen years old; the same person her mom, sisters, and best girlfriends have been seeing. If that's the case, read this tip to her. This isn't about loyalty, it's about reinforcing what the care provider says and making a well-informed decision as a couple. The worst thing that will happen is that you'll realize you already have the best care anyone could ever want.

THE BOTTOM LINE:

If your caregiver feels threatened by you getting a second opinion, he's not a caregiver who is being *loyal* to you.

Common Complications:

(Source: www.4women.gov)

Gestational diabetes is a form of diabetes that usually occurs in the second half of pregnancy.

SYMPTOMS: Extreme thirst, hunger, or fatigue (but usually no symptoms). Also, a blood sugar value of 140 mg/DL or greater on a diabetes test.

DIAGNOSIS: The oral glucose tolerance test.

TREATMENT: Most women can control their blood sugar levels with diet and exercise. Some women with gestational diabetes or women who had diabetes before pregnancy need insulin shots to keep blood sugar levels under control.

Hyperemesis gravidarum (HG) is severe nausea in the first trimester that can cause malnourishment and dehydration in some women. HG keeps pregnant women from drinking enough fluids and eating enough food to stay healthy. Many women with HG lose more than 5 percent of their pre-pregnancy weight, have nutritional problems, and have problems with the balance of electrolytes in their bodies.

SYMPTOMS: Severe constant nausea and/or vomiting several times every day for the first three or four months of pregnancy.

DIAGNOSIS: If you think your partner might be vomiting excessively, call the doctor who will check to see if she's dehydrated, which can be dangerous for her and the baby.

TREATMENT: Many women with HG have to be hospitalized so they can be given fluids and nutrients through an IV. Usually, women with HG begin to feel better by the 20th week of pregnancy. But some women vomit and feel nauseated throughout all three trimesters.

Urinary tract infection left untreated can spread to the kidneys. This can cause premature, or early, labor.

SYMPTOMS: Pain or burning when urinating; pain in lower pelvis, lower back, stomach, or side; shaking, chills; fever; sweats; nausea, vomiting; frequent or uncontrollable urge to urinate; strong-smelling urine; change in the amount of urine; blood or pus in the urine; pain during sex.

DIAGNOSIS: Urine test.

TREATMENT: Antibiotics, usually three- to seven-day course of amoxicillin, nitrofurantoin, or cephalosporin.

Placenta previa is a condition in which the placenta (a temporary organ joining mother and fetus) covers part of or the entire cervix. Placenta previa can cause severe bleeding usually at the end of the second trimester or later.

SYMPTOMS: Painless vaginal bleeding during the second or third trimester. In many cases, there are no symptoms.

DIAGNOSIS: An ultrasound exam.

TREATMENT: A diagnosis after the 20th week of pregnancy, but with no bleeding, requires cutting back on activity level and increasing bed rest. If bleeding is heavy, hospitalization is required until mother and baby are stable. If the bleeding stops or is light, continued bed rest is required until baby is ready for delivery. If bleeding doesn't stop or if preterm labor starts, baby will be delivered by C-section.

Preeclampsia is pregnancy-related high blood pressure. It can also be called toxemia. Preeclampsia usually occurs after about 30 weeks of pregnancy.
SYMPTOMS: High blood pressure (usually around 140/90); protein in the urine; swelling of the hands and face; sudden weight gain (1 pound or more a day); blurred vision; severe headaches; dizziness; intense stomach pain.
DIAGNOSIS: Blood pressure test; urine test; evaluation by a doctor.
TREATMENT: The only cure is delivery, which may not be best for the baby. Labor will probably be induced if condition is mild and woman is near term (37 to 40 weeks of pregnancy). If a woman is not yet ready for labor, her doctor may monitor her and her baby closely. May require bed rest at home or in the hospital, until blood pressure stabilizes or until delivery.

Premature or preterm labor: This is when a woman goes into labor after 20 weeks, but before 37 weeks of pregnancy.
SYMPTOMS: Contractions, either painful or painless, any time during pregnancy, that occur more than four times an hour, or are less than fifteen minutes apart; menstrual-like cramps that come and go; abdominal cramps with or without diarrhea; dull backache that may radiate around to the abdomen; increase in or change in color of vaginal discharge; constant or intermittent pelvic pressure.

DIAGNOSIS: Monitoring of uterine contractions by wearing an elastic belt around the waist that holds a transducer or small pressure-sensitive recorder. Can be worn at the doctor's office, in the hospital, or at home.

TREATMENT: Lie down with feet elevated; drink two or three glasses of water or juice. If symptoms do not subside within one hour, contact your doctor. May require medications called tocolytics or magnesium sulfate to stop contractions.

Ectopic pregnancy is a condition where the fertilized egg implants outside the uterus, usually in the fallopian tube.

SYMPTOMS: Slight, irregular vaginal bleeding that often is brownish; pain in the lower abdomen, often on one side, and can be followed by severe pelvic pain; shoulder pain; faintness or dizziness; nausea or vomiting.

DIAGNOSIS: Blood tests; vaginal or abdominal ultrasound exam (screening that uses high-frequency sound waves to form pictures of the fetus on a computer screen); laparoscopy (surgery to view the abdominal organs directly with a viewing instrument).

TREATMENT: Because the embryo of an ectopic pregnancy cannot survive, it is removed surgically; or the woman is treated with an anticancer drug, methotrexate, which dissolves the pregnancy.

Placental abruption is a condition in which the placenta separates from the uterine wall before delivery. This can deprive the fetus of oxygen.

SYMPTOMS: Vaginal bleeding during the second half of pregnancy; cramping, abdominal pain, and uterine tenderness.

DIAGNOSIS: An ultrasound exam.

TREATMENT: When the separation is minor, bed rest for a few days usually stops the bleeding. Moderate cases may require complete bed rest. Severe cases (when more than half of the placenta separates) can require immediate medical attention and delivery of the baby.

Mastitis is an infection in the breast that can happen during pregnancy or breastfeeding.

SYMPTOMS: Soreness or a lump in the breast accompanied by a fever and/or flu-like symptoms; possible nausea and vomiting; yellowish discharge from the nipple; breasts feel warm or hot to the touch; pus or blood in the milk; red streaks near the area. Symptoms could come on severely and suddenly.

DIAGNOSIS: Evaluation by a doctor.

TREATMENT: If symptoms are not relieved within twenty-four hours of the following steps, see a health-care provider (you may need an antibiotic). Relieve soreness by applying heat (heating pad or small hot-water bottle) to the sore area. Massage the area, starting behind the sore spot. Use your fingers in a circular motion and massage toward the nipple. Breastfeed often on the affected side. Rest. Wear a well-fitting supportive bra that is not too tight.

Tip #14
MISCARRIAGE TIP: Skip This One Unless You Need It

If you are in your first trimester and don't want to read about complications—just skip this. I'm serious. There's no reason to read it unless you're dealing with it. I included this tip in case you need to read about it. Just know that this tip is here and it's available on the next page to check out if you want to read it. If not, skip ahead to the next chapter on page 81.

THE TIP:

Being strong means sharing with her that you're hurting too. Don't hold it inside or it will come out in other places.

THE STORY:

Our first pregnancy went just as planned. Everything went well. During the next pregnancy, we lost the baby at 22 weeks. I got pregnant again but lost that next baby at six months.

For a good month, I cried. It was a long process. At first, everyone asked if we were both okay. Then the concern for him subsided and it was all just me. While I had as much time as I needed to grieve the loss, he had to go back to work. His body was at work, but his brain was still trying to deal with this. He spent so much time watching me and being helpful for me that he didn't have an outlet for his feelings. He's deeply personal and has a "never let you see me sweat" attitude. He always wants to be strong for the both of us. His strength during this time in our lives didn't come from bravado—it came from a place of "She's having such a hard time that if I sit here and cry, she will be a mental case. I need to be strong for her."

I cried for months. Meanwhile, I noticed that he started to change. He would snap at other people over things he never snapped about before. He was impatient and not himself. The emotions had to go somewhere—he needed an outlet. What ends up happening in a lot of marriages with a pregnancy loss is that if a couple doesn't communicate, the wife starts thinking the husband doesn't care and that he isn't devastated or upset. He buries his feelings. Then the couple grows apart and the marriage suffers.

Thankfully, we never got to that point. After noticing his short fuse, we talked about his feelings. We cried together. He needed to talk about it, and I needed him to talk about it. Not discussing it doesn't change anything. Talking about it together is what makes it better. And now we have three beautiful children. As time moves forward, this part of our life becomes smaller and smaller, but it's also the part that proved to me that I married the very best man.

> —*Jami, sons 6 years and 7 months,*
> *daughter 26 months*

✻ ✻ ✻

If you're grieving the loss of a pregnancy, the words on this page won't take away the pain. Grieving is a deeply personal process. What I want to communicate is that there is a community of people who understand and have been there before. As many as 25 percent of pregnancies end in miscarriage. Most occur in the first trimester. Many end before the pregnancy is detected. Miscarriage is nature's way of ending a pregnancy that wasn't healthy. There's not much anyone can do to keep this from happening. It's a natural part of the pregnancy process. You just don't hear a lot about it because people tend to keep it quiet, but it's extremely common and normal to a large degree.

Should she lose the pregnancy, one common reaction is for your partner to feel guilt and shame—as if she did something wrong. Reinforce that this miscarriage is nature's way of protecting life and ensuring a baby is healthy and able to thrive. This isn't about what she did or didn't do; it's about nature. Blame nature. There's no shame or guilt.

Once the sadness lifts, you'll likely get pregnant again. And plan on having a healthy child. Once enough time passes, this loss will fade to the back of your mind and become a distant memory. This may be hard to believe when the loss is all you can feel and think about, but all the dads I spoke to promise that it will pass.

Another issue that needs to be addressed is the number of couples who lose a child before birth and then lose their relationship. If there's ever a time to talk and have open communication, this is the time. She needs to know that you are feeling some sense of loss. She needs to know you're grieving too. She needs to know that you're connected. Women need you to be there. And not only do they need to see and feel your sadness, it will help you to get beyond this.

See, as the expectant father *you* aren't the one people worry about after the miscarriage. It's all about her, "How is *she* doing? How's *she* feeling? How's *she* recovering?" Very few people think to ask about you after the first week or two. Managing your partner's health and emotions, the family's emotions, and your own are a lot to handle. And for a lot of guys, you don't get much time to grieve the loss. You have to go right back to work and continue life as if nothing happened. If you're struggling to move beyond the loss, find a pregnancy forum online and share your thoughts. Lean on others who have been through this. Talk to a grief counselor who specializes in miscarriage.

When it comes to sharing the information with family and friends, do it sooner rather than later. Ask the people you shared the good news with to share the sad news with anyone they've shared with. You want to avoid having someone come up to you or your partner and ask about the baby. If you need guidance, talk to your spiritual leader, the social worker in the hospital, or a professional caregiver who specializes in preterm loss. You don't need to handle this alone, and you shouldn't pretend to be strong and have all the answers. Your feelings are just as important as hers. Reach out and lean on the community that's out there. Visit the discussion forums on www.DadsPregnant .com and share your thoughts. Please just know that you are not alone. In fact, there are millions of people who have been there who now have beautiful families. The pain will ease—trust that it will get better.

THE BOTTOM LINE:
Tell her how much you're hurting too. Grieve together, feel the loss together, and then, when you're ready, make more babies together.

3

THE BABY'S DEVELOPMENT

This Part Has Pictures

Welcome Expectant Fathers to the week-by-week guide.

The following information is a supplement to information you will receive during "reading time." Reading time is when your pregnant partner reads to you about what's happening with the pregnancy. Reading time is not an optional time. It's a mandatory week-by-week update of what's happening with the baby.

Depending on how much information your partner decides to share, you might hear references to sore nipples and various food analogies. The sore nipples are self-explanatory (hers, not yours). The food references help give you a sense of the size of the baby or your partner's uterus—one week it's a pea, then a grapefruit, then a cantaloupe, and then a watermelon (that's a big kid). Not paying attention can be interpreted as not caring. The challenge is that reading time can take place at inopportune times (Game 7 of the World Series, bottom of the ninth, bases loaded, team down by three runs). But no matter what else is going on, not listening means not wanting to hear about your unborn child, thus turning you into an AA (accidental asshole—see Tip #17). So along with reading time, I will provide you with a guide to read on your own time to help you understand the different stages.

On the following pages, you will find a quick reference guide with pictures to show you what's happening inside her. This section includes the development of the baby and the 40 weeks of pregnancy (yes, more like ten months). If you're looking for a more in-depth medical look at pregnancy, check out the *Mayo Clinic Guide to a Healthy Pregnancy* book. Online you'll find helpful guides at WebMD.com, BabyCenter.com, and iVillage.com. You can also pick up one of the pregnancy guides in the bathroom or on her nightstand to get more information.

The following pages should give you just enough information to enable you to impress her. For example, when the baby's hearing is fully developed by week 26 you can be like, "Only say nice things to me—the baby can fully hear you this week." That will impress her (or piss her off, turning you into an accidental asshole—see Tip #17).

WEEK 1

She's not *really* pregnant. In fact, the first week of pregnancy is a nonpregnant week. The reason we start counting from this week is because it's just not possible to know the exact date of conception. So, to calculate the due date, the first day of her last period is considered the first day of pregnancy. In a way, all women are fake pregnant from the time of their last period until they ovulate. It's not until the egg gets fertilized by the sperm that she is *really* pregnant.

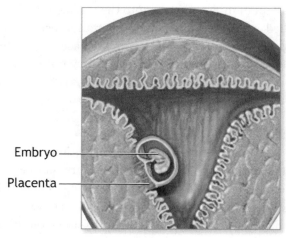

Embryo

Placenta

✽A.D.A.M.

WEEK 2

She's still not *really* pregnant. I know, it sounds like a bunch of crap, but conception doesn't occur until ovulation occurs (that should occur sometime during the second week). That said, this is the week the sperm should fertilize the egg and trigger the beginning of the real pregnancy. When conception happens, two of the forty-six chromosomes that make up your baby's genetic code will meet each other. Because the female egg is always an X chromosome, the male sperm determines the sex. A sperm carrying an X means you have XX, or a girl. A sperm packing a Y means you have XY, or a boy. A sperm carrying a Z means you've discovered a new species of baby.

Once the egg is fertilized it will make its way down the fallopian tube and settle into the uterine wall. This is called implantation. Once implantation occurs, the pregnancy hormone begins to release. It's this hormone that will enable your pregnancy test to blink, form an X, form a line, or announce *pregnant* (never seen a talking one).

WEEK 3

Now she's *really* pregnant. Congratulations. No one can tell she's pregnant, but things are happening inside her. It's a 24/7 of things happening. The fertilized egg is rapidly dividing into cells. First 2, then 4, then 8, then 16, then 32, then 64…you get the idea. Eventually all these cells form the blastocyst. The blastocyst is what attaches to the uterine lining (called the endometrium). The area where implantation takes place will become home to the placenta. (This is the organ that acts as the base to the baby and filter from baby to mom.)

3.5 weeks

✿A.D.A.M.

WEEK 4

You still may not know you're pregnant. If your partner has tingling or aching in her breasts (and you're not holding them) it's the hCG (a pregnancy hormone) which is also telling her body to stop releasing eggs and keep the uterine lining from shedding. The switches turning her body into a temple of new life will continue to flip as she goes into baby-making mode. At this point the pregnancy tests with the super-early detection might detect the pregnancy. Then again, they might not. It's not until the days following her expected period that the tests will be conclusive.

WEEK 5

This is the week she misses her period and the week you'll hear the news (assuming she tells you). This is also the week you become a lot less important. As for the baby, things are starting to take form. You're now the proud father of an embryo, and a heart is starting to beat. The embryo continues to make its way into the uterine lining. The neural tube is forming (this becomes the spinal cord and brain). The heart is forming. Also, the placenta is starting to develop. The placenta is an amazing organ that attaches to the uterus and acts as a conduit of nourishment from mom to baby. (Some people will cook it or bury it after the birth.) As for mom, she needs to watch what she eats—no blue cheese, bologna sandwich, or sushi platter with a raw egg dip to celebrate the pregnancy. If you have a cat, don't let her handle the poop. (Congratulations, that's now your job.) The litter can spread toxoplasmosis (a bad, bad thing for pregnant women).

WEEK 6

The brain and nervous system are taking shape. The beginning of the eyes and ear canals are forming. The baby's heart should start beating in regular rhythm at this time. The digestive system, respiratory system, and small buds that will become arms and legs begin to form. All this is happening and the kid is just an eighth of an inch long.

WEEK 7

The big development this week is that facial features are becoming more distinct. There are also hands, digestive organs, and lungs. An umbilical cord is now formed. This will give you something to cut once the baby is born. The mucus plug forms this week. It seals off the uterus from the rest of the world (and that's why sex isn't a problem unless your doctor says otherwise). Beyond the plug, early pregnancy signs may be surfacing (see Chapter 5).

7.5 weeks

✿A.D.A.M.

WEEK 8

It's Bud time—genital bud time. The buds that will form your baby's business are forming. It's still too early to know what you're having, but it's something. There's also pigment in the retina, arms that can flex, longer intestines, and early signs of fingers and toes. Your partner will be feeling pregnant or at least like her pants are tight.

8.5 weeks

✲A.D.A.M.

WEEK 9

After everything that's been going on, your kid is about an inch long and not even a quarter of an ounce. The baby's head is the largest part of the body. Flaps of skin that will soon become eyelids form. Intestines, an anus, and testes or ovaries are also forming. The baby's movement might be visible through an ultrasound which should show that beating heart (roughly 150 beats per minute).

WEEK 10

Enjoy your embryo because next week, it will graduate and become a fetus. That's right—time really flies. (I remember when you had buds for arms....) At this point, the vital organs are formed. The tail is gone. (Yes, it had what looked like a tail.) Testes, if present, begin producing testosterone. Fingers and toes begin to separate. The baby looks like a baby. As for your partner, she should have seen her doctor by now. Encourage her to ask the doctor questions. If she can't talk to her doctor, then find a new doctor.

10 weeks

✾A.D.A.M.

WEEK 11

Your fetus is around 2 inches long. That said, there's a lot packed into that 2 inches (yes, if you had a dime for every woman that told you that). The placenta is growing at a rapid pace to keep pace with fast growth happening over the coming weeks. Other than that, the ears are moving to their final location and the head keeps getting bigger. (It's half the size of the body.)

WEEK 12

This week you can raise your glass to little fingernails and toenails forming. Shout hooray for the vocal cords. With new working kidneys, your kid will now be able to pee on him- or herself. Mom's body is pumping more blood than ever. This increased blood

12 weeks

✿A.D.A.M.

flow and hormones cause greater oil gland secretion—this is what may give your partner that pregnancy glow (although if she glows in the dark, she needs medical attention). And with that, she gets a glowing review for her first trimester.

SECOND TRIMESTER: The Baby's Development (Weeks 13–27)

WEEK 13

At this point the placenta is almost fully functional. Think of the placenta as a home base—it's the control panel and the umbilical cord is the hose that connects the baby to the base. The placenta supplies the baby with oxygen and nutrients, takes care of waste disposal, and produces hormones (progesterone and estrogen) that are vital for pregnancy. At this point in the pregnancy, the eyelids are fused, the vocal cords are forming, and the baby has thumbs that can go in his or her mouth. The face looks like a little person's face. The internal organs are starting to rev up and do their thing.

WEEK 14

Your kid might need a shave about now. But don't worry about these hairs. They're called lanugo and they're said to be soft and colorless (but there's no such thing as colorless). Lanugo will continue growing until about the 26th week, and it will cover the baby's entire body. Lanugo goes away before birth (and it's replaced with vellus hair). The lanugo helps protect the thin skin from the elements. The size of a 14-week-old fetus is about 1 to 2 ounces (45 grams). If you were to stand the baby up it would be 3½ inches from head to rump.

WEEK 15

For the most part, the body parts and organs are getting strong and growing. The eyes and ears are moving into their final position. The baby can move its body parts. Soon, the mom will be able to feel something moving. My wife didn't start feeling anything until week 19, but it can start sooner or later. The uterus will move higher up above the hip bones to make room for the baby to grow. If you have an ultrasound machine at home (not recommended), by this week you might be able to see if it's a boy or girl—depending on how good you are.

WEEK 16

It's a lot more of the same, but more movement is happening. First-time moms might not feel it yet, but soon the visitor inside will make his or her presence felt. The legs are longer than the arms—prepare for someone to play soccer with mom's internal organs as the baby can kick. Fingernails are present and growing. The baby now weighs around 3 ounces and measures approximately 4 or 5 inches from crown to rump.

16 weeks

✤A.D.A.M.

WEEK 17
The baby can suck, swallow, and blink. Fat is starting to form. The baby is the size of a grapefruit—and not a very heavy grapefruit.

WEEK 18
This is a big week. The baby's ears are in position and your kid might be able to hear. When you talk make sure you do it loudly. You're competing against whooshing blood, gas, a heartbeat, and any other noises

that might drown out the important things you have to say. The baby is about half a pound now.

WEEK 19
If it wasn't bad enough having a kid with a hairy body from head to toe, this is about the time when a white cheesy substance called vernix starts to form. This is more protection for the skin from the fluid in the amniotic sac.

WEEK 20
At the halfway point, your baby weighs in at roughly 9 ounces and is about 6 inches long. The baby is sleeping and waking as if it were a newborn. The uterus is around mom's belly button, which may pop out. The shifting and growing baby will put pressure on mom's lungs, kidneys, stomach, and bladder. But this kid's only half baked. There's a lot more that needs to be done.

WEEK 21
The baby continues to develop and organs start practicing. The amniotic fluid carries sugars that can be digested through the baby's intestines. The rapid growth slows down.

WEEK 22
As the brain and nerves develop, the baby becomes aware of new sensations. The baby might move around to test them. If the baby is a boy, then the testes

begin to descend. If the baby is not a boy, there won't be any testes descending.

WEEK 23
Bones continue to harden, and the baby is just over a pound (or just about the weight of a bag of peanuts at the ball game). Things are moving in the right direction—like fingers, arms, legs, and toes. If your partner goes into premature labor this week, the baby has a chance of survival with a lot of medical care.

WEEK 24
This is considered the week of viability. Still, a baby born this early wouldn't be going home with mom or dad for several months, assuming it can survive on its

24 weeks

✤A.D.A.M.

own. The lungs continue to develop and prepare for the next phase of life outside the womb. The baby can gain several ounces in muscle this week.

WEEK 25
Your partner will feel the baby moving around a lot. The spine is forming. The ears are working and the nostrils begin to open. The uterus is about the size of a soccer ball, and it will get much bigger soon.

WEEK 26
The baby weighs between 1½ and 2 pounds by now and is approximately 9 inches long crown to rump. Brain waves for listening and seeing begin to kick in. At this point the baby should be able to hear you loud and clear.

26-28 weeks

✿A.D.A.M.

WEEK 27

Start saying good-bye to the second trimester. The baby looks similar to how it will look when it's born, but much smaller. But it's growing fast. If the baby were to be born at week 27, it would have a good shot at survival outside the womb.

THIRD TRIMESTER: The Baby's Development (Weeks 28–40 or longer)

WEEK 28

It's now the third trimester. The baby is about 2 to 3 pounds (maybe heavier) and 10 inches long from crown to rump. The eyes will open, the eyelashes are growing, and there's hair growing on its head. You can talk, sing, or rap for the baby—it can hear you and recognize your voice. The doctor may check to see where the baby's head is resting.

WEEK 29

The baby continues to grow and kick. A normal rate is to feel at least ten kicks an hour. If your partner isn't getting kicked ten times an hour, that's something to discuss with your healthcare provider. They say the baby has a sense of taste by now, so your partner should check with baby to see what he or she wants delivered to the womb and at what time.

WEEK 30

The baby is now about 3 pounds and getting bigger. It will put on about a half pound a week for the next seven weeks. If your partner thinks the baby might have hiccups, she's right. It's common as the lungs practice breathing. Your pregnant partner might be having a hard time sleeping. Heartburn and constipation might also be a problem for her. Suggest that she sleeps on her left side. I'm not just saying that. Research has proven this is the safest side in terms of blood flow to her organs.

30-32 weeks

✼A.D.A.M.

WEEK 31

The baby continues to grow. The doctor may check the level of amniotic fluid. Too much or too little can be something to investigate. The baby is now peeing several cups of urine a day. The baby's reproductive system is getting in position. The lungs aren't ready to work on their own yet, but they're practicing.

WEEK 32

The baby is about 4 pounds and 11½ inches long crown to rump. The lanugo starts to come off. If the baby was born this week, it would have a very strong chance of survival. Everything should be working. But you still want to keep the baby inside (especially if the nursery is under construction).

WEEK 33

This week rapid brain growth is happening. Amniotic fluid levels are at their highest. Weight gain continues. Eyes can detect light so your partner should avoid walking in front of headlights when baby is sleeping.

WEEK 34

More growing—the kid's just getting bigger. While the lanugo is gone, the vernix (the thick coating) gets thicker. You might see this when the baby is born. (They don't show this in the movies.)

WEEK 35

This week the baby's goal is to gain weight and collect fat. This continued weight gain will make it harder to move. Soon the baby will start to look for larger accommodations.

WEEK 36

At 6 to 6½ pounds and 16 to 19 inches long, the baby might soon drop into the birth canal to prepare for delivery. The doctor will start checking the cervix to see if it's dilated. Refer to the birth section for specifics.

WEEK 37

When this week ends, the baby will be considered full term. Your partner should experience more vaginal discharge as her body prepares for delivery. Don't expect her to show you or tell you about this. The position of the baby is important. The baby's head should be pointed downward by now. A breech baby might mean you have to plan for a C-section.

WEEK 38

This week the baby could gain as much as an ounce a day. The weight is close to 7 pounds. The intestines are accumulating more and more meconium. This is what makes up the first bowel movement (it's like a black tar poop). Your partner might be feeling false labor contractions.

WEEK 39

The baby's getting lower in the birth canal and is almost here. The kid can barely move at this point. Your partner might not be all that steady either; as the kid moves downward, mom's center of gravity can be thrown off. If she works in a circus, no tightrope this week.

WEEK 40

This week you should meet your kid...or the next week or the next. The average baby is 7½ pounds and around 20 inches. But none of this is certain. Soon, all hell will break loose. That's covered in the delivery chapter.

4

THE MANY FACES OF THE EXPECTANT FATHER

Inside the Male Mind and Body

There are many faces that make up the expectant father experience. The following are some of the most common faces you might see reflecting back at you in the mirror at some point during the pregnancy. If you have something to add or feel a face is missing, please send me a note, so that I can include it in future editions. (Send to www.DadsPregnant.com.)

Tip #15

THE IN-AWE EXPECTANT FATHER: Words Can't Describe It (But I'll Try)

THE TIP:
It's a feeling like nothing you've ever experienced before.

THE STORY:
Seeing the baby come out of my wife was surreal and mind-numbing. The image was too much for me to comprehend—it was sensory overload. It wasn't until a few hours after the birth, when everyone had been taken care of, that I had a chance to hold my daughter. My wife was sleeping, and we were alone. That's when the switch was flipped. It was a feeling I had never experienced before. I was awestruck by the pregnancy, by the birth, and by the delivery. But the love a father feels for his child blew me away. It's a feeling that never goes away.

—Me, daughter 22 months,
21 weeks pregnant

* * *

We had a C-section, and I got to spend time with Jack before Emily did; it's not how I wished it. He opened his eyes and he looked at me, and I said, "Hi Jack." And he looked at me like he knew that was his name. It was the most magical moment.
—*Jeff (son 9 months)*

I thought of including a blank page for this tip because there are no words to describe the feeling of going through the expectant father experience. But a book with blank pages isn't a good book. So, here's my best attempt.

Being an expectant father will leave you in awe. It will excite, exhaust, intimidate, embarrass, intrigue, surprise, scare, shock, and delight you all at once. The adventure will stir untapped emotions. It will leave you feeling something you've never felt or experienced before.

It's as if there's something programmed into our DNA that's activated during this process. And when the switch is flipped and it happens, the world will change forever. It's an emotional state so powerful and all-consuming that there are no words for it.

Don't worry about not feeling it right away. It *will* happen, but *when* it happens will vary. It could be immediately after the birth, or an hour, a day, a week, or a few months later—but it will happen. It's not something you need to force. No matter the heaviness or happiness of the moments leading up to the birth, it will all be worth it. The adrenaline rush of fatherhood is better than any drug—once the initial surge

It's like a Darwinian switch flipped in my brain. I went from reluctant father to head-over-heels committed dad in a heartbeat.

—*Eric (daughter 15 months)*

I was in awe when I saw the ultrasound of our baby and the heartbeat—that is when I knew it was for real.

—*Kevin (18 weeks pregnant)*

subsides, the feeling lingers forever. It's what bonds us to the baby.

From conception to coming home, the whole journey is exhilarating, exhausting, and awe-inspiring. It's something you'll probably want to do again and again. And while you might in fact do it again and again, savor the first time—the first is a once-in-a-lifetime experience. Enjoy the adventure ahead.

THE BOTTOM LINE:
You won't believe what you see, hear, and feel.

Tip #16
THE REJECTED EXPECTANT FATHER: Embracing the URT of Fatherhood

THE TIP:
Sometimes even your smell will make her sick.

THE STORY:
One of my weird pregnancy symptoms was that I could not be touched, kissed, hugged, or held for weeks. I couldn't have him too close either. It got so bad that even the smell of him—you know the smell of a guy—made me queasy. It wasn't that *he* smelled, it was *his* smell. We didn't kiss for at least a month. This went on for weeks and weeks. I told him that it wasn't anything about him, but it still bothered him,

I could tell. I apologized whenever I told him to not hug or kiss me, but he looked hurt. After a while, he gave up trying and told me to tell him when he could kiss me again. Once it passed and I was able to smell him, things got better. I don't think he ever quite got it when it was happening. I felt guilty because I could tell I was disappointing him, but I didn't have any control over it.

—Samantha, son 11 months

✳ ✳ ✳

Over the years, I've uncovered an unspoken and universal truth that consumes so much of our time and energy. I call it The Universal Rejection Truth (URT) and it's the undeniable force of nature that says not everyone we want to appreciate, include, and desire us will always appreciate, include, and desire us. Millions will, but millions will not. There are an infinite number of URTs in nature. A few you might be familiar with:

- The Universal Rejection Truth of Dating and Relationships says that not everyone we want will always want us.
- The Universal Rejection Truth of Sales says that not everyone will appreciate, include, and desire our services.

It's one thing to have her tell you she's not in the mood, it's another to have her tell you that the idea of having sex with you is so far from her mind that the thought of it makes her want to vomit.

—Matt (father of two)

- The Universal Rejection Truth of Being a Student says that not every teacher you have will always appreciate, include, and desire us.

The most familiar and feared URT is The Universal Rejection Truth of Dating and Relationships. The URT of Dating and Relationship says that not every one we want to hold us, touch us, and spread love oils on us will always want to hold us, touch us, and spread love oils on us. Millions *will* but millions *will not*. You're probably thinking, "No shit, I know this already." The problem is that while most of us know this, most of us are stuck in a state of rejection denial. Rejection denial is a deep dark place where we refuse to acknowledge or accept the Universal Rejection Truth. Applied to the the world of love, we never give women (or men) we like permission to *not* like us. When we're stuck in a state of denial and we get rejected, we get angry, upset, or withdrawn. We take rejection so personally because we can't see beyond our own insecurities. We can't see a truth more powerful than us—that rejection isn't always about us, but about the laws of nature.

The Universal Rejection Truth of Expectant Fatherhood says that your partner might not always appreciate, include, and desire you during this experience. She might spend time with friends, family, books, her laptop, not kissing you, not having sex with you, and not taking care of you. Once the baby is born, it's only going to continue. You'll go from #2 to #3 (you moved to #2 when she was pregnant) in her eyes. This doesn't mean that she loves you any less; it means that nature has made her a mother, and this role requires her to place her pregnancy and her child in priority above you. It's normal, natural, and part of the process.

What makes it so hard is that all these changes can leave an expectant father more vulnerable and uncomfortable than ever before. Not getting the attention you're used to getting when more vulnerable than ever can make a guy withdraw or become resentful. Some guys look for attention from other women. Some become controlling. Some hang out with their own friends. Some get mean. Some become disconnected. But few of them talk to their partner and ask what they can do to be more involved or connected.

Here's the secret: Give your partner permission to reject you and understand that it's part of the process. Instead of taking it so personally and running away or resenting her, ask her what you can do to help her feel connected. Embrace the URT of expectant fatherhood and let her feel whatever it is she's feeling. Most pregnant women don't even realize what they're doing and how it affects us. Instead of taking the rejection personally, listen, talk to her, and find new ways to stay connected.

THE BOTTOM LINE:

It's not about you, but the URT. Fight it and it will tear you apart. Accept it and it will ultimately bring you closer together than ever.

Tip #17

THE ACCIDENTAL ASSHOLE EXPECTANT FATHER:
Good Guys Who Make Mistakes

THE TIP:

Even the most loving and supportive guys can be accidental assholes. Your partner will forgive you eventually. (Diamonds help speed the process.)

THE STORY:

My man was an accidental asshole on two occasions in a very short span of time. The first incident happened before leaving for the hospital. While my contractions were becoming increasingly more painful and regular, he decided that the best thing to do would be to TiVo the Bears game, so he wouldn't miss anything. Meanwhile, I was hunched over the kitchen counter and yelling at him to leave the house. By the time we got to the hospital, I was already at 4 cm. Once we arrived and settled into our room, he did it again. We were told during our Lamaze classes that our husbands need to be sure to eat while we are in labor, but absolutely *not* in the room. So, what did my husband do? The first chance he got, he went down to the cafeteria and got

During labor, right before the transition stage (really intense contractions), my husband realized that he had left the car at the curb in front of the hospital and left to move the car! I really missed his presence in the room while he was moving the car.

—*Anne (mother of four)*

himself a nice hot breakfast of eggs and bacon, which he proceeded to bring back up to the room and sit and eat in front of me because he didn't want me to "be alone." My husband was very supportive, but those weren't his best moments.

—*Jenn, daughter 2 years*

* * *

We've all been there before—and if you haven't been there yet, you will at some point in your relationship. We are all accidental assholes. The accidental asshole is a well-intentioned man who makes a mistake. It might be something you've said, done, or didn't say or do. Most often, it's made without ever knowing that we did something wrong. The best of intentions can yield accidental asshole results.

Some examples of classic accidental asshole moves:

- The loving father who buys his wife hot lingerie ten sizes too big after the pregnancy.
- The loving dad who goes to the doctor's appointment and thinks it's funny to make jokes about her weight.
- The caring dad who cooks his wife dinner and forgets to tell her that the salad has blue cheese crumbles.

I was flying home from Hawaii with my wife and our 3-month-old. Turns out that I packed the formula in the checked luggage and boarded a plane for a nine-hour flight! They had to stop the plane and return to the gate so we could get the formula out of the cargo area.

—*Isaac (father of two)*

- The dad who compliments his partner's new big boobs and calls them better and hotter than her normal boobs. (He also gets too excited and uses a slang word to describe her huge new breasts.)
- The loving father who tells his wife to suck it up when she's in the midst of her morning sickness.
- The expectant father who encourages his wife to avoid pain meds because he had a cavity filled without novocaine and it wasn't too bad.

It's important to note the difference between being an accidental asshole versus being an intentional asshole. An accidental asshole doesn't mean to upset his partner, and he feels genuine remorse when she gets upset. An intentional asshole purposefully disregards his partner's feelings and doesn't feel any remorse when she gets upset. In fact, upsetting her is often the goal (sick, I know).

While few of us are intentional assholes (upsetting our partners on purpose), we all will be accidental assholes at times. When it happens, don't try to explain it—apologize and admit that you didn't mean to be an asshole. To try and defend yourself just makes you a bigger asshole (and then you run the risk of being an intentional asshole). Embrace it and trust that all of us at some point will be one. Most of us are used to it. It's a bond that links all expectant fathers, husbands, partners, and boyfriends together.

Please share your accidental asshole moments at www.DadsPregnant.com.

THE BOTTOM LINE:
We're all accidental assholes. To deny it would be an asshole move, which would make you an intentional asshole, and that's the worst kind of asshole.

Tip #18
THE SCARED EXPECTANT FATHER: The Things Men Think, But Rarely Say Out Loud

THE TIP:
The idea of having a baby can be terrifying.

THE STORY:
We had planned to start trying to knock her up in May of last year. But right before then, I was suddenly struck with cold feet, and I told my wife that I wanted to wait to have children. I wasn't sure if I even wanted kids at all. I didn't feel ready, and I wasn't prepared to give up my happily selfish lifestyle. The truth was I was terrified. My dick-ish declaration sent my wife into a crying jag for days. Obviously, I soon saw the light— that no one is ever truly ready. You just have to jump in with both feet. Having a child was the smartest decision I ever made—an exhausting clusterf**k.

—Eric, daughter 15 months

✳ ✳ ✳

There will be moments when you get scared and ask yourself, "What the hell am I doing?" The idea of being a father will make your head feel like it's going to pop off your shoulders. Everything that comes along with being an expectant father can be overwhelming. It will hit you when you least expect it. You will ask yourself:

- Am I ready for this?
- Will I be a good dad?
- What if there are medical problems?
- How can we afford this?
- What if something happens to her during delivery?
- What if something happens to the baby?
- What if I pass out or can't be there for her?
- What if the baby doesn't look like me?
- What if my partner can't handle being a mom?
- What if I can't be a good enough husband?
- Why does she keep rejecting me?
- Why do I feel so out of control?
- Why do I feel so scared?
- Why is my partner so distant?
- Why am I so overwhelmed?
- Why am I so attracted to other women?
- Why do I feel like I just want to run away?
- Will I be as good of a parent as my parents?
- Will our relationship survive?

> Time at the gym is time for myself and a stress release. I need it and she understands and supports it. From what I hear, time for myself isn't something I'll have much of once the baby is born.
>
> —*Eric (28 weeks pregnant)*

• Why didn't anyone tell me about this?

Part of being a first-time dad means allowing yourself to feel all these things and knowing that you're 100 percent normal. You're allowed to feel reluctant, terrified, unsure, scared, out of control, or whatever else you're feeling. To not feel these things is to be an expectant father in denial.

Big life events will fill your head with big thoughts. If you're 16 and expecting your first, you have good reason to be terrified. If you're 26, 36, 46, 56, 66, 76, 86, 96, or 106 (106 is kind of old for kids) and expecting your first, you too have good reason. These feelings are what bonds us together. It's just that men don't sit around telling each other what scares them, and pregnant women don't necessarily want to hear what scares men. So, it's all a big secret. Now, the secret is out.

Instead of fighting it, or running from it with drugs, alcohol, addiction, or other women, allow yourself to feel it all *and* not have the answers. Talk to other guys who have been there and done it. Post an anonymous note on www.DadsPregnant.com. Find a positive activity as an outlet for stress (working out is perfect). If these normal thoughts start to interfere with your daily life, make an appointment with a therapist— there could be more going on (see Tip #29: The Not Happy Expectant Father). Whatever you do, be patient with yourself.

My prediction (based on hundreds of interviews) is that the moment you look into your child's eyes, the fear and anxiety will melt away. Yes, it's normal to feel apprehensive, to question yourself, to question your partner, to question the future, and to feel overwhelmed at times. But try not to let it freak you out too much.

THE BOTTOM LINE:
Feeling scared isn't a bad or weak thing—it's normal and natural.

Tip #19
THE "FIGHTING CHANGE" EXPECTANT FATHER: Life Will Change… But for the Better

THE QUESTION:
How do you prepare for dramatic change when you don't know what the dramatic change is going to be?

THE STORY:
At our age and having been married for five years, our life is set as far as being able to go out to dinner at 8:30, doing what we want, going on vacation every six months—but the realization is starting to hit me. There are a lot of things that scare me. I'm worried about things changing—mostly how we

There's a thought that birth will magically bring a couple together. But it is a profoundly stressful time that continues long after the baby is born. The solace was that we spent time building our relationship.
—*Todd (father 2 months)*

will change as a couple. What if that's all she can talk about? What if she becomes one of those women I see at lunch whose only work is spending the day with the kids? I don't want to be one of those couples who just talks about their kids to each other and when they're out with other people. We've always hated those people. I'm more religious than she is, and I don't want to argue about choices we make for the kids. I think back to all the things my parents did for me. My parents were great—they took us everywhere. What if I'm just selfish? What if I'm not like that? What if being a dad doesn't come naturally? What if I have to force myself to be that way? I'm not around a lot of little kids—I don't enjoy being around little kids. Will I learn to like being around kids? I'm not great with that stuff. I've never had an interest. You know what it is? I'm worried because a lot of my friends don't seem happy—they love their kids, but they don't love their relationship after having kids. I love our life.

—*Walter, 30 weeks pregnant*

* * *

Listening to guys talk to each other about having a kid can be depressing at times. It's mostly all about how "You have no idea how much things will change." They say it in a way that isn't hopeful or bright. The tone is serious and foreboding. They don't tell you about all the amazing parts of the change. They leave out that it's the most amazing, awesome, and worthwhile change in the world. They leave out the part that it's made life better. They leave out all the best stuff. And that's not fair.

But yes, the immediate change can be jarring. And it's largely because most people don't see it coming because up to now there hasn't been much to prepare you so you can anticipate what will change. The first 3 to 6 months are the toughest for a lot of guys—but it gets better, and better, and better. But you have to trust and know that it will get better. I'm telling you, if you want it to get better and plan for it to get better, it will.

Losing the life you love can be a sad thought. But what your life will soon become is something you will *never* want to change. Think about it like this: If life is great without a kid, assume it will get better with one. The things you fear losing will be negligible compared to what you will gain. Of course, parenting can bring up new conflict and it will change your dynamics as a couple, but if you've been able to handle problems in the past, you'll be able to work through them in the future.

The couples who feel disconnected and at odds are couples who have a history of problems or a gut feeling that something isn't right going into this. But even that isn't necessarily a bad thing if you're willing to discuss it. Having a child will not magically fix everything (it will only bring fundamental problems to the surface), but talking to your partner when issues comes up and planning for change can make all the difference in what happens next.

1. **PLAN FOR LIFE TO CHANGE**, but for the better. If you're constantly telling yourself the change will suck, you're inviting problems into your life. Plan for life to change for the better and it will.

2. **DON'T FIGHT IT.** It's like a hurricane rumbling into your world. Start building a stronger foundation with your partner so you can weather the storm. When the storm clears, life will be better—far better.

3. **BE PATIENT.** Be patient with yourself, with her, and with the baby. It can take a good year to get comfortable with all the changes. It's the biggest transition of both of your lives—it takes time to create a new rhythm.

4. **HELP YOURSELF.** Read, talk to other new dads, speak to a therapist on your own or with your partner, work out, and find a positive outlet to channel the emotions. There's never been a better time or reason to make changes and reach out for support.

5. **YOU'RE NOT ALONE.** If it sucked so bad, billions of people wouldn't be doing it again and again. It's not bad; it's great.

For more insight into "The Change" and putting together an "Action Plan" to help anticipate, embrace, and manage the changes ahead, flip ahead to Tip #92.

THE BOTTOM LINE:

You've just been shown the wrong previews. It's not a scary movie—it's more of a thriller or romance with a happy ending.

Tip #20
THE EDUCATED EXPECTANT FATHER: Enjoy This Book in the Bathroom

THE TIP:
Bathroom reading can keep you involved.

THE STORY:
The pregnancy wasn't too anxiety-provoking for me. I think what helped is that I did a lot of reading. I read her mom books and a couple of dad books. My wife also had a subscription to *American Baby*, and she would leave the magazines and other reading materials in the bathroom for me. She didn't pressure me to read them, other than leaving them where she knew I'd find them. It took me a while to figure it out, but the magazines all look alike and have the same articles because there are new people constantly going through the same experience. Reading helped keep me involved and up-to-date with the development of the baby. Sometimes, when we talked and she'd bring up

something about the development, she'd be surprised and impressed when I expressed some knowledge.

—Jeff, son 9 months

∗ ∗ ∗

However you got your hands on this book, I appreciate that you're reading it. Not only because it helps me afford diapers and a double stroller, but because it's something I wish I had the first time around. I know writing it has helped me the second time around (my wife is about 22 weeks pregnant now).

So much of being an expectant father is about facing the unknown and navigating through so many emotionally charged experiences, all of which are new. Facing the unknown and experiencing dramatic change can be naturally uncomfortable. Being an educated expectant father will give you enough of a baseline of what's normal and to be expected. If you know what's normal and expected, it won't be such a big deal when you see, feel, or experience something that's naturally uncomfortable (and so much of the expectant father experience can be uncomfortable).

For example, if you know that your partner will experience practice contractions (called Braxton Hicks) throughout the pregnancy, the first time she feels a contraction won't freak you out as much. Another example: Should she want you to have sex with her (a big hypothetical), you don't have to be afraid of poking the baby in the forehead because you'll know that the cervix is sealed tight (plus there's the amniotic sac protecting the baby). Likewise, when your partner sees something strange, feels something new, or experiences something weird, you can reassure her instead of escalating the situation.

By having a baseline of knowledge, you can get comfortable with the uncomfortable. And that means not overreacting, not having to be right all the time, and being a better listener because you're not spending your time worrying and internalizing the experience. Once you have a solid foundation of what's normal, the unknown isn't so intimidating. It just makes this whole thing easier to approach.

There are so many resources out there to help you along the way. This book is one. I've also included a number of titles at the back of this book. One in particular is *The Mayo Clinic Guide to a Healthy Pregnancy*. This amazing resource has great information should you want concise medical information. (Of course, you should always be able to talk to your caregiver.) Another resource is the Internet. *Beware*: Make sure the information you're reading is from a trusted source. There are a lot of crappy sites out there. My rule is that when reviewing online information, it has to be medically-reviewed information. The #1 bookmark for me is MedlinePlus (http://www.nlm.nih.gov/medlineplus/). Another trusted site is WebMD. At these sites you'll find links to trusted medical resources and credible sources (but always consult your caregiver). The Internet should never be your final destination to find answers; that's the job for your caregiver.

Other great sources of information are the pregnancy books for women. It's always interesting to see and hear how the information is being delivered to women. *The Girlfriend's Guide to Pregnancy* (by Vicki Iovine) is a classic that can give you a good sense of how women talk to women about these issues. *Belly Laughs: The Naked Truth about Pregnancy and Childbirth* (by Jenny McCarthy) is another. Also, check out her pregnancy magazines. They make for some riveting bathroom reading. Reading a few articles can keep you involved and part of the process. It might even help you get lucky. The more you know, the more comfortable you can get with the uncomfortable.

That said, there is such a thing as being too educated. Ignorance can be a good thing when it comes to complications or other less enjoyable issues. If your caregiver isn't concerned about complications, don't spend too much time reading about them. And really, if you don't like any of the topics in this book because you'd rather not know, just skip them or rip out the pages (actually, ripping out the pages would be a sign of bigger anger issues—reread Tip #18). There's enough to worry about without becoming consumed with what can go wrong. Assume everything will be alright. There's no reason to read about anything other than the good parts (unless you're writing a book about it).

THE BOTTOM LINE:

Help other expectant fathers become educated expectant fathers. Please share your stories via www.DadsPregnant.com or via email at Harlan@helpmeharlan.com, subject "Dad's Pregnant." Thank you.

Tip #21
THE ALWAYS ON-CALL EXPECTANT FATHER: There's No Escaping…

THE TIP:

Sometimes she doesn't want answers—she just wants you to answer.

THE STORY:

One day when my son was a couple months old, he was going crazy at home. I was at work and my wife must have called me three times—over and over again. I can't always answer my phone during work because I'm…working. But she kept calling. When I finally picked up she was wigging out because the kid was crying. She tells me, "I can't take it anymore. What's his problem? I can't do this!" I told her, "It's gas." And then she starts screaming, "It's NOT gas." I make a suggestion and she yells at me. I can't talk because I'm working. And then it ends up being my fault that he's crying. When I come home at night he's sleeping and she's back to herself. Everything a guy does is his fault. I'm used to that as a cop—everything is our fault.

—Mark, son 2½, daughter 6 months

✳ ✳ ✳

Something has happened. There's no escaping. Our generation is facing a new issue that no man has ever faced before. Cell phones, email, and text messaging have made it easier than ever for women to tell us everything that they're feeling, thinking, and experiencing on a second-by-second basis—especially pregnant women and new moms.

Not only will you be physically going shopping, she will call you when she's shopping. She will call you when her mood swings. She will call you when an idea pops into her head. She will call you when the baby is crying. She could call you more than she's ever called you before. This might be something you love or it might be something that you find to be too much, but you're always on call.

When your pregnant partner emails, calls, or texts with something on her mind, you need to pay attention or you will see many of the different faces of the pregnant woman appear. How to set boundaries when you are so easily reachable is a challenge. As available as you were before the pregnancy is how available you need to be after the pregnancy. Not taking a call because you don't want to talk means that you don't want to support her—at least that's how she might interpret it. If you can't talk, explain that you care about her and support her, but you have to do whatever it is that you're doing. The biggest mistake is dismissing her, blowing her off, or pretending you're unavailable. If you pick up and she's in the midst of an outburst, then listen and wait until the outburst cools. If you do attempt to be helpful and find yourself in the line of fire, resist firing back. You can be right and she can be wrong without her knowing you're right and she's wrong (see Tip #46).

If you find that you can't get away from the constant communication and need a break, make sure you have a place in your life where you can find some space. Designate a time in your schedule when you aren't available—going to the gym is perfect. You can also find space attending a sporting event, driving, hanging out in windy and noisy places, or traveling to places with no cell phone reception, like underground subways, mountain peaks, or a developing country. There's nothing wrong with giving yourself a short break every now and then.

THE BOTTOM LINE:

You can try to run out of battery charge, you can hide in voicemail, but she will always find you...and that's okay because she might be in labor and in need of a helping hand.

Tip #22
THE DEMOTED EXPECTANT FATHER: Standing in the Shadow of Her Belly

THE TIP:
It's like being on the bench when you used to be on the starting line.

THE STORY:
When she was pregnant, I didn't care that she was the center of attention. I'm not one to get jealous of that. After our son was born, it was not what I expected. She breastfed him so there wasn't much I could do. She would feed him and console him and I'd stand around. I would try to hold him, but she would tell me there's not much I could do for him. And then, when I did hold him, he would cry and I couldn't do much for him because he wanted to eat. She was taking care of him, and he wanted to be with her. I didn't think this was what fatherhood would be like. I thought I would be a lot more involved. I felt like I was a player waiting on the sidelines—waiting to be called into the game. While I waited, I walked the dog a lot.

—Phil, sons 1 month and 2½ years

✳ ✳ ✳

How are you doing? Seriously, I might be the first person to ask you this question.

Once the test turns positive, you drop a rung on the ladder of importance. You move from #1 to #2 and there's nothing you can do about it. If you are married, it's kind of similar to what happened during the wedding planning process. Once she was engaged, the wedding became the #1 priority. After ten months of planning, all you wanted was for things to get back to normal so you could live your life together. The big difference between the love train and the baby train is that once the wedding train pulls into the station, we move up to #1 again. After she pushes out the baby, we move down another rung to #3 (we are behind the baby and our partner).

There are two phases that make up the dad demotion:

- **Phase 1**—From when the pregnancy strip turns positive until the baby is born.
- **Phase 2**—From birth until his or her first birthday.

During this time period, you are no longer the center of your partner's universe. And it's not just her universe, it's the universe of friends, family, and co-workers. It's rarely, "How are you doing?" It's usually, "How's she doing?" or "How's the baby doing?"

> I think my boyfriend was used to being #1 in my life. Then he was booted to #2 when the baby came and I really think that was and still is hard for him sometimes.
>
> —*Gina (daughter 4 months)*

Once the baby is born, a mom's maternal instincts take over—and that's when things can get even more challenging at home. The vast majority of first-time moms don't have a firm grasp on what's happening with the baby or with themselves. This is true of most first-time dads too, but moms tend to be the primary caregivers, so they have primary control. Not knowing what's happening can be uncomfortable, and uncomfortable people tend to want to be in control. This happens with a lot of new moms during and after pregnancy. They want to be in *total* control. It can be her way or no way. Fighting it means fighting a losing battle. After doing things wrong so many times, it's just easier for a guy to just not try to get involved. But knowing this is coming can help make it easier to handle. Instead of letting this new dad demotion deflate you, make it motivate you to stay that much more involved.

Being #3 can suck at times—no question about it. But fighting it can make it suck that much more. It can even make some guys look for attention from the wrong places (see the box about what *not* to do). What expectant fathers need to understand is that being demoted is a normal and natural part of the process. And new moms can be controlling and protective, which can make it worse.

> I wish I had told my husband, "You will always be the first person in my life, but you may be put in the back of the line a few times. It won't be long before you are in the front of the line again."
>
> —*Yasmin (mother of two)*

The thing is that most of them don't even realize what they're doing. When it's happens, talk about it with them—bring it up (never in the midst of a fight). If you can't talk to your partner about it for whatever reason, then reach out and find someone you can talk to. Just avoid reaching out to a hot neighbor or sexy coworker (bad choices). After a year or so, the sun will shine and the belly will go away. And so will the shadow you've been standing in.

How to get attention when demoted:

- Attend as many doctor's appointments as possible.
- Share pregnancy books with your partner (and read hers).
- Shop with your partner for baby stuff (buy her maternity store gift cards—*don't* guess her size).
- Plan activities (**NOTE**: Pregnant woman can't ride roller coasters).
- Go on a getaway (a trip is a great way to stay connected).
- Document the pregnancy with photos and video (of her belly).
- Journal your feelings (keep a blog).
- Talk to other guys about things you're feeling.
- Talk to a therapist, health professional, or spiritual leader.
- Go online and be a part of this forum: www.DadsPregnant.com

How not to get attention when demoted:

- Confide in a hot coworker.

- Confide in a hot neighbor.
- Confide in a hot female friend.
- Confide in strippers (not hot ones are excluded too).
- Confide in hot online strangers.
- Confide in a hot ex (or any ex that still wants you).

THE BOTTOM LINE:

The dad demotion is normal and to be expected. If you need attention, don't look for it from a stripper (unless your partner is a stripper).

Tip #23
THE GETTING FAT EXPECTANT FATHER: Proving Your Love One Nacho at a Time

THE TIP:

She'll get full faster than before. Don't eat what's left on her plate; it will make you fat.

THE STORY:

We wanted to eat out as much as possible before the baby came, thinking that a newborn baby would be noisy and not good at restaurants (not true by the way). So we'd go out to eat, and my wife would eat part of her meal but become full because her stomach was small. So I'd eat mine and hers, effectively super-sizing every meal! The food was there and I could not avoid eating it. Portion control was the major issue. I gained a total of 20 pounds during the pregnancy. I felt fat—like the stereotypical overweight dad at little league games. My wife didn't say anything because she always thinks I'm thin. I figured that I would just take it off. Once the baby was born, I went on NutriSystem (Dan Marino's diet). We also realized our gym has a baby-sitting service, so I got a personal trainer and worked out. It took me a few months to take it off, but it's gone.

—Jay, daughter 21 months

✳ ✳ ✳

They're not called paternity clothes—they're called fat pants.

I didn't actually give birth to my daughter, but I ate like I was going to. When my wife had our baby, she gained 35 pounds and afterwards lost 20 of them in one day. I gained 15 before the delivery and another 5 pounds after it. I ate during the whole pregnancy and delivery. (I put down my sandwich during the final push.) When she craved it, I ate it.

There is actually a name for the sympathy weight a father gains. It's called "Fat Dad Syndrome." No, actually it's called couvade syndrome, and there's been clinical research to show that some men will also have increased levels of hormones and exhibit similar symptoms as their pregnant partner (but remember, you can never say, "Me too!"). Part of couvade syndrome can be phantom weight gain. It's common to put on 5, 10, or 20 pounds. One theory is that a man who exhibits similar symptoms to his partner communicates to her that he's connected and in it for the long haul. (There are hints that our primal relatives share a common approach. In a study cited by *Nature* magazine, male monkeys also gained weight during their counterpart's pregnancy.)

Here's how it happens: When a woman who typically eats salads and healthy foods starts craving ice cream, pizza, tater tots, and mac and cheese, a loving partner will join in the action to be supportive (and because it tastes good). He'll eat it all just so she doesn't feel alone. After joining in for nine months, that supportive partner can get fat—love handles, an extra chin, a bigger pair of pants. Two pounds a month is all it takes to show the love.

If you have a history of weight gain or are struggling with weight issues (emotional eating), prepare to gain some weight and struggle. As your family grows, so do your responsibilities (and pants size). Food can be a crutch, and there's going to be a lot of it around you. If your partner watches what you eat (i.e., she tells you not to eat so much crap), don't expect her to keep tabs on you. She'll be too busy watching her own belly to watch yours grow enormous. This means you will have to cut yourself off. Going on a diet before you need it is a good idea.

Interestingly, the second- and third-time dads I interviewed were less likely to gain. As a first-time dad, the only thing I lost once the baby was born was sleep. Knowing this, I can't afford to gain any more weight the second time around because once the next baby is born, there will be even less time to go to gym and take it off (unless you have a gym at home).

Now, if you happen to lose a lot of weight while your partner is gaining a lot of weight, don't make a big deal about your weight loss. *Never* offer her your old pants. That's one way to guarantee she'll *not* be getting in your pants (see Tip #57: Guide to Pregnant Sex). Stay active, make working out part of your routine, and start a diet before you need it. Her pregnancy is not a license to eat like a pig.

THE BOTTOM LINE:
If she asks you why your bottom line looks so big, tell her it's because you love her.

Tip #24
THE DO-IT-ALL EXPECTANT FATHER: Making Sure It Gets Done in Time

THE TIP:
Do all the stuff you're leaving for the last three weeks earlier because she might get put on bed rest.

THE STORY:

Having her on bed rest was the worst. She was diagnosed with high blood pressure (preeclamspia) and wasn't able to get out of bed—no preparing meals, nothing other than showering and going to the bathroom. I was in charge of working and getting ready for the baby. I would leave at 7:30 in the morning and come home at 6:30 at night. When I came home I had to make sure she got dinner, I had to keep her spirits up, entertain her, and then I had to set up the nursery—cleaning, shopping, getting diapers, bottles, and all that stuff. Her cell phone bill that month had to be about $600 more. She didn't move. It was a mutual appreciation—she was incredible through it all. She was put on bed rest six weeks before her due date, but it turned out to be three weeks because she went into labor early. I couldn't wait for the baby to born. As soon as she delivered, her blood pressure dropped and her weight dropped (she gained 90 pounds). It was like night and day. The couple of days when she was in the hospital were the best. It was the first time in weeks I was able to stop moving.

—Jason, daughter 4 months

* * *

We have to do a lot. Not a big surprise. You're probably doing something right now for her—perhaps reading this book because she made you do it (or not). There's a lot more she'll want you to do. I'll get to this in the Nesting Pregnant Woman tip, but this one is more about setting a timeline to get it done.

What surprised me while researching this project was how many guys had pregnant partners who were put on bed rest. There are different kinds of bed rest (all take place in a bed, but some are more restrictive). Should she get put on bed rest, there's no resting for you. Even if she isn't put on bed rest, she might need to rest in bed more as the due date approaches. She might not be able to do everything she wants to do. That's probably one reason she's so insistent on getting it all done months before you think it needs to get done. Maybe deep in her psyche she thinks she might be unable to do it. If she can't do it, you'll be left doing more than you're already doing—which I assume is a lot.

But whether it's bed rest, regular rest, or the baby coming early, you'll want to be prepared. Whenever your due date is, subtract a month and make that the date by which *everything* needs to be done. If you find that she can't do what she used to do (because of exhaustion or bed rest), technology can be your friend. When it comes to stocking up on supplies for the baby, order them online and have them shipped. When it comes to groceries, order them online and have them delivered. When it comes to cleaning, get a service to come once every two weeks during the final months.

When it comes to things like new construction and home improvement projects, *do not plan on her being available during the last month of the pregnancy*. The due date is about as reliable as the contractor finishing on time. Get it done early. The worst thing that will happen is that you will have extra time to hang out with your pregnant partner and play with her belly.

THE BOTTOM LINE
Plan on the kid coming a month early and plan on the contractor being a month late.

Tip #25
THE PROTECTIVE EXPECTANT FATHER: Watching Out for the Guy in Seat 25D

THE TIP:
If you have to yell at her to stop moving the couch, yell politely.

THE STORY:
We were in the midst of moving when all of a sudden she started lifting things. My wife has always been one to do it her way—even if her way involves moving 60-pound boxes and risking her own health or the child's. That's exactly what she did. She would push around the couch to get to the boxes. And she would do it with

me right there. She knows that I would do it for her—
I'm the one who schleps. I'm sitting there with able
hands and a pregnant woman is moving things. There
was nothing I could to do stop her. So, I yelled at her
in the nicest way a guy can yell. She got mad—I swear
it was a polite yell, but she kept lifting. She moved a
huge couch to move the 60-pound boxes. That's how
the third trimester started.

—*Chuck, son 2 years*

✳ ✳ ✳

You're going to want to protect her from bad drivers,
strangers rubbing her belly, dangerous food that will
mess her up, pain, aches, herself, weirdos, and
overeager family and friends who won't leave her
alone. Here's how to protect her the right way:

FROM RUDE PEOPLE

Not everyone will yield the right of way. Not everyone
will open doors. Not everyone will give up their seat.
Some people will argue with her. Some people will
upset her and make her cry. The way to exert control
over the things you can't control is to control yourself.
When it happens, you'll get pissed. But no one understands. The people acting like this are most often
people who don't know she's pregnant or don't know
what it's like to have kids. Give people permission to
be stupid and selfish.

FROM BELLY TOUCHING

For some reason, people will think your partner's pregnant belly is there to touch. Women will touch. Men will touch. Old people, young people, friends, family, coworkers, classmates, and strangers in elevators will reach out to touch it. In addition to getting her a T-shirt that says, "Touch me, I taze you," and a custom-made button that says, "No touching my belly please," encourage her to set boundaries. If someone touches her, she has every right to tell that person that she's uncomfortable. The "uncomfortable" word is the least confrontational.

FROM ORDERING HIGH-RISK FOOD

Other people at the dinner table might criticize you or give you a hard time when you ask a server at a restaurant if the milk is pasteurized or if the Caesar salad dressing has raw eggs or if the meat is cooked all the way through—ignore them all. You have every right to ask questions. Instead of attacking the people who harass you, educate them. If they keep riding you, give yourself the label of the most loving and protective father. If "annoying" is part of that label, that's not a bad thing to be (see Tip #7 for a refresher).

FROM HERSELF

Pregnant women will assert their independence at times. No one wants to feel helpless. Protecting her from herself can be another issue. Whatever you do, try to avoid yelling at a pregnant woman when she does something she shouldn't do. It's never cool to yell at a pregnant woman. It just provokes her to yell back, cry, or make you look like a big bully. A less confrontational way is to tell her that you're really upset about something—then ask her for advice on what you should say to get her to listen. Have her tell you how to talk to her. If you do yell at her, apologize. If after week 20, also apologize to the baby for yelling at mommy (he can hear ya).

FROM THE ACHES AND PAINS

Giving birth can be painful (so I hear), and there's nothing you can do to stop the pain. You can only help manage it (or ignore it). Helping her with breathing, counting contractions, acting as a strong advocate, finding the best care, communicating her birth plan to the team, being involved, staying informed, and holding her hand throughout the process is the best way to protect her. Just being there is doing so much.

FROM RANDOM VIOLENCE

It's a fact that women are the most vulnerable when pregnant. No pregnant woman should be out alone after dark if it can be avoided. In addition to things like pepper spray, a taser gun, or a whistle, consider having her take a self-defense class. Still, a pregnant woman is a target, and she needs to be reminded to be extra vigilant. And unfortunately, sometimes it's the partner who is doing the harm. (If you ever have feelings of wanting to hurt her or feel trapped, please get help.)

FROM FAMILY AND FRIENDS

It doesn't seem like family and friends would pose a problem, but they can get in the way. It could happen before the baby is born by calling over and over again to see if she's gone into labor yet. It could happen during labor with family walking into the delivery room. It could happen once the baby is born with everyone coming over. You need to be the buffer to help her be comfortable, rested, and happy.

THE BOTTOM LINE:

You might want to protect her, and you can do a lot, but you can't always be there to be the buffer. She also needs to protect herself.

THE GUY IN SEAT 25D:

The other day we were boarding a three-hour flight from Chicago to California. I had an aisle seat one row in front of my 20-week pregnant wife and 22-month-old daughter. They were in seats 25E and F (a middle and window). I was in seat 24D (the aisle seat in front of 25D). We asked the guy in 25D if he would trade with me. He said, "No." His buddy was sitting across the aisle from him. It took me an hour at 34,000 feet to let it go. He had to be in his forties or fifties—I can't imagine that he has kids because no father would separate a man from his family and leave his pregnant wife to take care of a toddler.

Tip #26
THE CALM EXPECTANT FATHER: So Cool She Might Think You're Cold

THE TIP:
Sometimes being too calm can cause her to get even more upset.

THE STORY:
I'm probably more calm than my wife wants me to be, but that's just how I am. I don't panic because someone needs to stay calm and be in control. During the first pregnancy she was put on bed rest at 30 weeks, and our son was born a month early. This pregnancy we've been to the hospital twice and everything has been fine. At around 25 weeks, my wife was feeling some discomfort and called the after-hours line. We were sent directly to labor and delivery. They hooked her up to the contraction monitor, but not much was happening. Then, most recently, at about 30 weeks, she felt some contractions and we went to the hospital. This time the contractions showed up on the monitor, but they weren't cause for concern. Again, they sent us home. When I tell her that everything will be all right, her emotions take over, creating a minor flare. I just don't get scared. I tend to think everything will be okay, but sometimes she doesn't want to hear it. There are some people shitting their pants (pardon

my language), but I saw my friends do it and realized it doesn't have to be so difficult. She sometimes feels that I'm disconnected because I'm so calm, but I express my excitement and concern in different ways. When good things are happening, I get excited. When the not-so-good things happen, I need to be mentally in control. So, I don't panic.

—Jon, son 25 months, 31 weeks pregnant

✳ ✳ ✳

There *is* such a thing as a calm expectant father. I'm not one, but there are guys out there who are calm throughout the process. Your personality might be calm or you might be responding to and trying to balance out a partner who is anything but calm.

And that's really what this tip is about—while you might be calm, she might be anything but calm. She might think your constant calmness is constantly annoying. Your level of calmness and cool nature could be causing her to become anxious and irritated. The idea that she's freaking out and you've *never* been more relaxed just might not have a calming effect. I mean really, as a guy, you have every reason to be calm. It's not like you're the one who is going to have to push out a 7-pound baby through your vagina.

Being so calm might also make her think you're not concerned. I mean, it's easy for you to be calm because *you* don't have to feel completely out of control when you start gaining weight (which you might actually do), getting swollen, getting sick, and having a kid yanked out from between your legs. She may think that, clearly, if you're this calm you must not be seeing her point of view or understanding what she is feeling.

How could anyone caring be so calm?

The calm expectant father can stay calm, but he needs to make sure to validate her experiences and not negate her. It's the difference between telling her that her aches and pains are nothing and holding her hand and massaging her aches and pains away. It can take work to show her that you're connected. If she feels pain and she's concerned, she'll want you to be concerned. You can be calm and concerned, but she needs to know that you feel her pain.

I agree, if you're going to spend your time and energy worrying, better to spend it on things that are worth worrying about. In most situations, there isn't anything to worry about, and you might have no idea where her emotions are coming from. But if she's worried, let her know that you understand and think that her feelings are valid.

THE BOTTOM LINE:

Remember, it's easier for an expectant father to be calm because men don't have to push a living person through a tiny opening in between our legs.

Tip #27

THE TIP:

Never tell a pregnant woman you're tired too. They don't want to hear it—especially when they're in labor and haven't slept.

THE STORY:

I had insomnia with all three of my pregnancies. I was completely exhausted. My husband would wake up in the morning after a full night's sleep and proceed to tell me how tired he was, as if I was supposed to feel bad for him. To top it off, my first labor was long and hard. It lasted 22 hours. He slept 16 of those 22 hours while I was in painful labor. When he woke up, he told me how tired he was after his 16-hour nap.

—Joann, daughters 4 years and 2 years, son 8 months

✳ ✳ ✳

This one took me a while to figure out—not that part about knowing that pregnant women hate it when men echo their symptoms, but

I want to feel like I'm the only one in the world who's pregnant. I know other women have been pregnant before, but when I'm feeling something, I want to think I'm the only one.
—Ellie (39 weeks pregnant)

figuring out why it pisses them off so much. See, when she tells you that something bothers her, she wants attention and wants to be taken care of. When you tell her that you feel the same thing she's feeling that means *you* want attention and *you* need to be taken care of. And she has too much going on to worry about that.

If your partner is complaining that she has a headache, don't say, "My head hurts too." If your partner is tired, don't tell her how tired you are too. If she says she's nauseous, don't be nauseous too. When she complains about aches and pains, don't talk about your aches and pains (even if you're a professional football player). If she says that she can't sleep at night, don't tell her how you can't sleep either. If she talks about her big belly and stretch marks, you can talk about *your* big belly and stretch marks, but only in an attempt to make fun of yourself (weight jokes about her are *never never never never never* funny—she might laugh, but she'll kick your ass later).

As much as she loves you, she doesn't want to hear about your ailments. This doesn't mean she doesn't care about you, it just means that she's not interested in hearing about it at that very moment. Chalk it up to the Universal Rejection Truth of being an expectant father (see Tip #16). But don't take it personally.

She told me that she was constipated when she was 38 weeks pregnant. I told her I was constipated too. She told me that she didn't give a sh*t.
—*Matthew (father of two)*

If you need to complain, preface your complaint by telling her that you know she doesn't want to hear about it, but you wanted her to know so she could understand why it's too hard for you to do something. It might take cooking dinner and vomiting in the pan for her to realize that you're not feeling well either. Or if you need to complain, call up your mom or your buddies. Tell them that you feel like sh*t and that no one seems to care. You can also post a note online and get it off your mind. I know man, you're tired. Being an expectant dad is exhausting. Your feet hurt, your head hurts, you're exhausted, you're stressed, you're fat, you have bad skin, you're nervous about the future—I'm here for you man. I know. I understand. I care. We all care—you just can't tell your pregnant partner about it.

THE BOTTOM LINE:
By saying "me too," you make yourself the center of attention and send the message that you want to be taken care of. But pregnant women don't want to take care of you. So take care of yourself. Grab some Tylenol or some Tums and stop stealing the spotlight.

Tip #28
THE EMOTIONALLY RESERVED EXPECTANT FATHER:
You Gotta Let It Out, Man

THE TIP:
Even the smallest expression of affection can mean so much to her.

THE STORY:

We had just returned from the hospital and his parents came over. I was soooooo tired! The simple fact that they were in the room upset me. I love his parents so much! We get along great, but for some reason, at that moment I couldn't handle being around them. I went into the bathroom with the excuse that I had to go and just cried! After a few minutes, my husband came in and just hugged me. He stared into my eyes and told me that everything was going to be okay. He said I was tired and took me upstairs and laid down with me so that I knew everything would be okay. I absolutely love that memory. He was so sweet when he stared into my eyes. He isn't affectionate, so that took a lot for him to treat me that way!

—Nancy, daughter 15 months

✳ ✳ ✳

I try to be the typical guy filled with machismo—the type that doesn't cry. After she told me though, I was instantly filled with all types of emotion that I couldn't help it. I picked her up and gave her a big hug (I'm about a foot taller) and started to tear up a bit while grinning from ear to ear and laughing.

—Kevin (3 months pregnant)

Definition of the emotionally reserved expectant father: A man who rarely expresses his true feelings in a manner that will reveal a softer side, but loves his wife/girlfriend/partner as much as the most emotionally effusive, loving, and expressive men.

This tip isn't about changing anyone; it's about pointing out that pregnant women who have emotionally reserved partners need more, and sometimes it's hard for these men to pick up on this. Less expressive does not mean less loving; it just means less likely to express loving feelings as frequently as a pregnant woman might need to see it, hear it, and feel it.

Sure, if you're emotionally reserved, your pregnant partner knows who she's with, but who she is while pregnant and who she was when you first met her are different. While she might have been fine with this nonexpressive thing before, pregnancy can change this. She's going to need more—however much it is that you can express.

Whatever you did to show her you loved her before the pregnancy, do it five to ten times more often during the pregnant months. Pregnant women have different needs, and they had no idea how much more affection they would need once they became pregnant. If your style isn't to talk openly about your feelings, then don't say it, just show her. Attending birth classes, getting flowers, buying maternity clothes (or a gift card), attending appointments, enlisting the help of a doula, encouraging her to have a friend participate in the delivery, inviting her family to stay with you during the delivery, giving pregnancy massages, and asking if you can do something around the house (and meaning it) matter.

> I wish he knew how much it means to me for him to *act* excited about the baby. I know he is excited, but it would be nice if he showed it more often.
> —*Amanda (18 weeks pregnant)*

Make sure she knows it and feels it on a regular basis. If you can't say it, find a way to express it. There's no such thing as making your pregnant partner feel too loved—not feeling loved enough is the problem. At least that's what the women I've interviewed told me again and again.

THE BOTTOM LINE:
Emotionally reserved doesn't mean less loving, but pregnant women need you to step it up.

Tip #29
THE NOT HAPPY EXPECTANT FATHER: When You Know Something's Not Right

THE TIP:
If you sense deep in your gut that there's a problem with your relationship, don't wait for it to get better. Talk about it and attempt to face it together if you want to have a chance of staying together.

THE STORY:
I got married and had kids at a very young age. After we had our daughter, I thought it would get better. When we had our second son, I knew it was too late. I never felt like my feelings were validated. Looking back, I should have been more vocal about my beliefs and feelings. I was always waiting for things to get

better, for her to adjust, but it never happened. The blame I put on myself is that I allowed society to dictate what I should be doing instead of listening to my gut. It's like telling a guy who's thirty-five that he's supposed to be married, so he goes out on a date looking to get married as opposed to finding someone he has something in common with. It has to be right. I've realized being a couple is not about forcing a relationship to work, but finding a real relationship that's about mutual respect, love, and comfort. The rest of it falls into place. It would have been helpful, less painful, and less expensive (divorce is costly) to figure this out the first time around.

—Nick, sons 6 months and 2½ years

✳ ✳ ✳

It's challenging enough to be in an unhappy marriage, but to be in an unhappy marriage and expecting is the ultimate inner struggle. You want to be happy, but there's this nagging feeling something isn't right.

Change can trigger a lot of emotions and old nagging problems ultimately surface. It might take months or years, but they will surface. There's this fallacy that having kids will bring a couple who is drifting apart

Suddenly he discovers a love of community theater that didn't exist prior to my pregnancy! It is such a passionate love that it takes him away from attending Lamaze classes with me! Needless to say, we are divorced now.

—Michele (mother of one)

MEN AND POSTPARTUM DEPRESSION:

According to a study published in the *Journal of Pediatrics*, "Approximately 14 percent of mothers and 10 percent of fathers suffer from moderate or severe postpartum depression resulting in undesirable parenting practices and limited parent-infant interaction." Postpartum depression (PPD) is more than just the "baby blues." These are feelings of deep and prolonged sadness, emptiness, and sense of failure and can include thoughts of suicide. The study continued to mention that depressed fathers are less likely to engage with their children and that pediatricians should screen the parents for symptoms.

closer together. It doesn't really work like that—at least in the long run. Core beliefs can clash. New issues and conflicts can develop. And if you have a history of dealing poorly with conflict, it's bound to happen again.

It's understandable—having a kid means that the dad is often demoted (see Tip #22). First it's the pregnancy that takes priority. Then it's nurturing the baby and the lack of sleep. Everyone is exhausted, overworked, and dealing with huge changes. Life amounts to standing in the shadow of her belly waiting for things to get better. It's easy to give her time to find balance. It's easy to ignore the problems and get wrapped up with your child's life. It's easy to push the problems aside. And then it's easy to get pregnant again. And then you have two kids and the same problems come up. This can go on for years. But the problems will not go away until you face them. Pushing them aside just makes it more painful in the long run.

If you weren't happy with your relationship before she got pregnant, don't expect that life will be better after the baby is born. It might be great for a few months, but old problems don't go away. I'm not saying this to depress you; I'm saying it because you can work to bring yourself closer to your partner before it's too late. The alternative is to do nothing and let this drive a wedge between you. The more disconnected you feel now, the greater the risk of falling into a depression and/or looking for attention from someone else.

If it's too hard to talk to her while she's pregnant about the issues that are troubling you, there's nothing wrong with you finding someone you can

MEN AND POSTPARTUM DEPRESSION: (Contd.)

But considering only a small percentage of men attend doctor's appointments and symptoms surface two to three weeks following delivery, identifying men who need help is that much more challenging. If you think you might be suffering from PPD, contact your local hospital or a postpartum hotline and inquire about referrals for men and treatment programs available in your community. Also check out Postpartum Support International at www.postpartum.net. If you're having thoughts of suicide and you need immediate help, call 911 or the following hotline: (800) SUICIDE. (For more on PPD, see Tip #49.)

Infidelity is a common problem when it comes to expectant fathers or new dads. Some reasons why it happens with such regularity include:

- Rejection can wear you down (see Tip #16: The URT of Fatherhood).
- Having to be responsible for so much is too much.
- The fantasy of a life without so much responsibility and stress is attractive.
- The marriage was already bad and beyond saving.
- People you date are less likely to make demands on you (freedom).

Learn to recognize these warning signs before you make a mistake you'll regret.

talk with. If you find yourself unhappy to the point of having dangerous thoughts (see sidebar), seek professional care. Face it. Once you have a child, you will forever be connected to this person. For that reason alone, it's worth the work to try to fix what's broken. Even if you think it's too late, until you try to fix it you'll never know. Besides, couples counseling is far less painful and costly than dealing with a separation and divorce.

THE BOTTOM LINE:

It's worth trying to make your relationship better. Face the truth and work through it sooner rather than later. Denying or avoiding problems only creates more problems.

Tip #30
THE TWO FOR THE PRICE OF TWO EXPECTANT
FATHER: Twins, Triplets, Quadruplets, Quintuplets…

THE TIP:
Do not fight it. You'll have to devote 90 percent of your time and energy to your family, and nothing could be more difficult or rewarding. It might start off being exhausting, but it will get better.

THE STORY:
We had no idea what was coming. The first thing that popped into my head was complete shock. Then it was, "How are we going to pay for this?" Then it was, "How difficult will it be with two?" We never anticipated this. The pregnancy was hard on my wife. She was sick and on antinausea medication for the first five months. At 29 weeks, she went into premature labor and delivered the babies via C-section. We took one of our daughters home after ten days. The other one came home after four-and-a-half weeks. Having twins was something no one could prepare me for. Basically for about six months, I got by on four or five hours of sleep and drove 35,000 miles making sales calls. It took a toll on my sex life, work life, and personal life, but I would *not* give it up for anything. Two and a half years later, I look back at what we went through and love it—I would do it all over again.

It was the hardest—I went from partying to having no time for myself or my wife, but we came through it. And trust me, it only gets better. My daughters are best friends. They can play with each other and don't need as much attention. We have more time to be a couple and to be ourselves. Now, it's the best.

—Kenny, twin daughters 2½ years

* * *

Congratulations! You're twice as lucky. Two for one sales, buy one get one free, and get the second at half price have never been so relevant (I don't think insurance companies offer coupons—check your Sunday newspaper). In a couple of years, you will have two or more kids who are best friends. If you're only looking to have two kids, pregnancy will be one and done. It's just that for right now, twins means twice the work and half the sleep. But I'm told, as hard as it might be, it's so cool to have two little kids once they get over the, "I can't do anything for myself" phase.

Carrying multiples means a shorter pregnancy (37–39 weeks is the target), more doctor's visits, additional risks (preterm delivery, gestational diabetes, and high blood pressure are just a few of them), more weight gain (about 35–45 pounds is

Everything was a challenge—having two babies cry at the same time, no sleep. The best advice I have is to make sure the husband gets out of bed as much as his wife does. It should be equal.

—Angela (twin sons 24 months)

the target), more hormones (and a higher risk of postpartum issues), possible bed rest, possible C-section, and two college tuitions in about eighteen years. (That's not fair, but you have eighteen years.)

The most important piece of advice is to encourage her to have a support network in place before the babies arrive. Do it sooner rather than later. Once the babies are born, she's going to be too busy to do much for herself. Start early so you can have a network waiting for you.

Because caring for multiples can be all-consuming, simple things like going out to lunch or going to the mall with the babies is going to be harder for her. She might feel isolated, overwhelmed, or alone. Most women with multiples don't have a lot of people surrounding them who have had multiples or are pregnant with multiples. When it comes to relating to the experience,

TYPES OF MULTIPLES:

- IDENTICAL TWINS: The result of a single fertilized egg dividing into separate halves and continuing to develop into two separate but identical babies. These children are genetically identical.

- FRATERNAL TWINS: The result of two eggs being fertilized by two separate sperm. They are no more alike than any siblings born to the same parents.

TYPES OF MULTIPLES: (Contd.)

- SUPERTWINS: Triplets, quadruplets, or quintuplets. Triplets occur in approximately 1 in 7,000 to 8,000 births; whereas quintuplets are likely to be born only 1 in 47 million births.

(Source: kidshealth.org)

having a network of friends (even online friends) can make a difference.

Ask your caregiver to suggest a support group. Also check out the National Organization of Mothers of Twins Clubs, Inc. (NOMOTC). The website offers this description, "NOMOTC is a network of more than 450 local clubs representing over 25,000 individual parents of multiples—twins, triplets, quadruplets, and more. NOMOTC promotes the concept of mutual support for parents of multiples. Opportunities for self-help and emotional support are provided through local and statewide meetings." (Visit NOMOTC at www.nomotc.org.)

When it comes to being a dad of multiples, the physical, emotional, and financial demands can mean working longer and harder than ever before. You might not be able to be there for your family as much as you want. This is one more reason to enlist as much support as possible—from family, friends, and care-givers. Investigate enlisting the help of a night nurse to help out for the first few weeks at home. (Babies typi-cally wake up every two and a half hours to feed, but twins aren't always on the same cycle, which means you could be getting very little sleep.) Consider hiring a baby-sitter once a week—not so that she can leave, but so she can shower and have a few minutes to herself. If you're depending on parents to help, ask them for as much time as possible to help you with the transition to home. And about home—preterm twins often must stay longer in the hospital after birth before growing strong enough to make the trip home. Once you get home, watch out for signs of postpartum depression in your partner. There's research that points to women who have had multiples as being more vulnerable to PPD.

BIRTHING CLASSES:
When registering for birthing classes, find out if there's a special class for couples expecting twins. If there isn't a special class, make sure your instructor is aware that you're expecting multiples so he or she can offer you additional instruction and information.

THE BOTTOM LINE:
Two-for-one college tuition—now *that* would be a great thing! Maybe in eighteen years.

Tip #31
THE ADOPTIVE EXPECTANT FATHER: All the Joy without the Morning Sickness

THE TIP:
Once the waiting part is over, we start to forget about waiting. Like any painful experience, your brain has a wonderful way of forgetting the awfulness. I blame it on sleep deprivation.

THE STORY:
We've adopted two children. For the first one, we waited seven months until we were matched up with the birth mother. We set up a nursery with the bare essentials and kept the door closed. Because my wife wasn't going through the physical experience, it was largely a surreal bureaucratic experience that was emotionally wrenching. The waiting process was the worst part. Once our daughter came home, other than the lack of sleep, it was terrific. At that point, my experience wasn't that different from that of a biological father. Having a wife who hasn't given birth is quite nice—this is an advantage of the adoption process.

You're not looking after a child with a wife who physically feels like she's been hit by a bus.

—*Andrew, daughters 20 months and 33 months*

ANOTHER STORY:

It was a Wednesday, and the social worker called me at work. She's says, "So, what are you doing?" I answer, "Just working." She's continues, "Anything important today? Because a baby was born on Monday." I asked her, "Have we been chosen? Is it a boy or a girl?" She says, "It's a boy and we want to know, can you get him today?" My husband was in New York and would be there for the next three weeks. I told her, "I can be there." Then I called my husband with the news. That's how we had our second child.

—*Linda, daughter 5 years, son 2½ years*

✳ ✳ ✳

Welcome adoptive fathers.

It's very important to include this tip because adoptive fathers go through so many of the same experiences as biological fathers. And, at the core, being a father, biological or adoptive, is a shared experience in which we all have much more in common than not.

That said, there are differences. Not dealing with a pregnant partner is one of them. There are also

ADOPTIVE FATHERS AND BIOLOGICAL FATHERS: A SHARED EXPERIENCE

- We share the unpredictable nature of expecting.
- We share the dramatic change our lives undergo.
- We share the exhaustion we feel once the baby is born.
- We share the emotional roller coaster.
- We all want to be strong for our partners.
- We share the shock and awe of being a father.
- And we share the love a father feels for his son or daughter.

grueling questions like: Will the birth mother choose your family? When will it happen? Will she sign over her rights to the adoptive parents once the baby is born? Should you have an open adoption (and meet the mother)? Should you have a closed adoption (where you don't meet)? What will the baby be like? Just like a biological father, until you live it, you don't know it.

Clearly, if you're going through adoption, there is support and a community to reach out to. With 120,000 parents going through adoption every year (according to the Child Welfare Information Gateway), there are people you can lean on to guide you. But when it comes to the other core issues (see sidebar), I hope this book is helpful in how it touches on some of the universal themes.

One important issue that adoptive parents alone have to deal with is that in order to have a child, you are judged and investigated. People judge you and trust that you have what it takes to be good parents. On the other hand, biological fathers can be completely unfit buffoons and still have a child. The truth is that none of us know what we're doing, and we all trust that we're fit to be parents, but adoptive fathers have already proven they are capable. And that's a good thing to remember, especially during that first night home when the baby is crying and you're thinking, "Can I do this?" Biological parents have to blindly trust that we can do it. You know you can do it—at least professionals who have judged you believe you can.

THE BOTTOM LINE:
We are all fathers: husbands, boyfriends, and partners.

5

THE BODY OF THE PREGNANT WOMAN

Like Puberty All Over Again

Each woman's physical experience with pregnancy is unique and unpredictable. Her body no longer belongs to her or to you. Each day can present a new ache, pain, or malady. Some women have little discomfort; others can't ever get comfortable. However your partner's body changes, always remember: Never touch her breasts without first getting permission. That can be bad, very bad.

Tip #32
THE BODY OF THE PREGNANT WOMAN: Like Puberty All Over Again

THE TIP:
How would I describe how it feels to have a pregnant body? Three words: *out of control.*

THE STORY:
Everything has expanded—my chest (not so terrible), butt, thighs, and of course, belly. Getting dressed in the morning and finding that I've outgrown my favorite clothes is a daily occurrence. Since the third month, there's been a new ache every day. Sometimes it's my lower back, sometimes it's my hip, other times it's a leg cramp. I never know what to expect. The relaxin that my pregnant body is producing makes my joints looser and less stable. I get weird cramps in my pelvic bones when I exercise or move around too much. It's easier to strain different parts of my body, especially when I'm carrying around my two-year-old. My belly button can be seen through my winter coat. It looks like someone drew a line down my stomach with a magic marker. I can't lift and do as much as I could before I got pregnant, which is seriously annoying. Sleeping is no fun at all. I wake up with hip pain and I can only lie on my side. I'm a total stomach sleeper,

so I'm tossing and turning all night when I'm not waking up to go pee. I definitely get that this is all for the good of the baby growing in my belly, but please— I'm only in the fifth month. I'm worried about what's going to happen to me over the next four! Don't get me wrong, I love that I'm having another baby. I just like having more control over how I look and feel.

—Stephanie, daughter 22 months, 22 weeks pregnant

She's going through a hulk-like transformation (she might even turn green). Her mind and body are in the midst of a second puberty all over again. There's no such thing as being too dramatic when your mind and body are out of control. And this brings me to the one reason why men don't get pregnant. If guys got pregnant, they would be so uncomfortable that they would just kick everyone's ass.

It's remarkable how women can deal with so much and still find time to work, take care of us, and be loving. The good news here is that some pregnant women experience very few of the most uncomfortable symptoms; but truthfully, most will experience some of them and additional symptoms not yet recorded in the medical journals. (Please send those to me via www.DadsPregnant.com.) Here's what she might contend with:

HER RAGING HORMONES

It's like the fourth of July inside her. There's an explosion of estrogen, progesterone, and relaxin pumping. You might think she's just being dramatic, and she might very well be dramatic. (Don't tell her to stop being dramatic or you'll only create more drama.) There's a reason for the drama. Her hormones are soaring at levels never before experienced and her moods might swing. See Tip #42 for more information.

HER EVER-EXPANDING UTERUS

In order to accommodate the baby's growth, the uterus will grow. As it expands it will push everything out of the way. Think of walking through a crowded bar on the way to the bathroom. The people in the way are the other organs in the body. She's going to get very uncomfortable. And she'll probably have to go to the bathroom a lot (but not in crowded bars).

The uterus is amazing. It gets a thousand times bigger during pregnancy (bigger than most expectant fathers' stomachs). It goes from a 2-ounce balloon that can hold less than a half ounce, to 2½ pounds in weight—big enough to hold the baby, the placenta, and about a quart of amniotic fluid. When the baby leaves, the uterus shrinks back to its original size.

HER INCREASED BLOOD LEVELS

Your partner's blood volume will nearly double during pregnancy (blood levels increase roughly 45 percent).

This leads to an increased heart rate and a new look for her with swelling in various places.

EXTREME EXHAUSTION
Pregnant women get tired—more tired than any man can possibly understand. Their bodies are working harder than ever before, pumping more blood than ever before, and carrying more weight than ever before. On top of the physical changes, there's the emotional exhaustion. It will make you tired just reading about it. (More in Tip #39.)

FEROCIOUS HUNGER
Pregnant women need more calories and more food—about 300 extra calories a day. Some pregnant women go from zero to starving in about one second. If she's hungry, feed her (make sure you move your hands quickly when feeding a pregnant woman). Whatever you do, do not question her hunger or food choices. (See Tip #35.)

MORNING SICKNESS
The surge of hormones during the first trimester can send some women into a constant state of nausea. Some women will have it for months (even the entire pregnancy), and others won't have it all. (See Tip #34.)

TERRIBLE GAS (HERS, NOT YOURS)
Pregnant women get constipated, gassy, and bloated. It can get so bad that they can't control it. Does a pregnant

woman get a free pass when passing gas? More about this one in Tip #36.

LARGE SENSITIVE BREASTS (HERS, NOT YOURS)

In a matter of days, her breasts will possibly double in size. Don't get too excited. These are not intended to feed your fantasies, just the baby. (See Tip #33.)

VAGINAL DISCHARGE AND HEMORRHOIDS

She's always had discharge, but now she has more of it. As for hemorrhoids, they're just another one of the gifts that can come with pregnancy. Increased blood volume and pressure on the veins in the rectum make this a common occurrence. (See Tip #37.)

SNORING AND LEG CRAMPS

One reason she might be so exhausted is that it's hard for her to sleep. And with the snoring, leg cramps, and constant trips to the bathroom, it might be hard for you to sleep too. (See Tip #40.)

DEPRESSION AND MENTAL HEALTH ISSUES

Depression can be triggered by all the hormonal changes. It can happen during and after pregnancy. The good news is that it's something that can be treated. See Tip #49 for more details.

OTHER FIRST-TRIMESTER ISSUES
- Shortness of breath

- Constipation (be sweet, get her interesting reading material)
- Mild cramping (especially after an orgasm, should you be so lucky to be part of this)
- Excessive saliva (makes for wet kisses)
- Heartburn (makes for restless nights)
- Itchiness (she might need a foot or belly scratch)
- Stretch marks (about half of women will get them)
- Occasional bleeding (never comforting)
- Frequent urination (keep this in mind while planning road trips)
- Headaches (it's not just an excuse, it's just incredibly common)
- Body aches, lower back pain, swollen ankles

THE BOTTOM LINE:
It's understandable why she might resent you at times. Being pregnant can be a huge pain in the ass (see Tip #37).

Tip #33
THE BIG-BREASTED PREGNANT WOMAN: You Can Look But Don't Touch (Without Asking)

THE TIP:
Pregnancy boobs are a catch-22 for many men. All of a sudden, you have a real banquet but you aren't allowed to feast.

THE STORY:

They were the untouchable treasure, the forbidden fruit. Hers were extremely large. There was no getting near them because they were always in pain, and in turn, I was always in pain. I would try to get close to them on a daily basis, and she would deny my efforts on a daily basis. I had a name for them, but if I share that name she'll read this and kill me (and I'll never touch any boobs). I never complained or got to the point where my attempts were more than good-natured. I didn't resent her large pregnancy boobs, but I prefer her pre-pregnancy boobs because I could touch those. I would advise other men to avoid touching and not complain about it. You can't complain because at the end of the day it's not you pushing an 8-pound something out of an orifice. Although, a nice pushing present might help a guy get within arms' reach.

—Larry, daughter 2½ years

* * *

Expectant fathers will discover that pregnancy breasts are far different than pre-pregnancy breasts. Pregnancy breasts tend to take on the personality of the pregnant person attached to the breasts—they can be unpredictable, sensitive, and irritable at times. They can

> Her boobs got huge. She went from a B cup to a D cup. And she didn't yet look pregnant. They were like natural nonsilicone instant breast implants. Those were fun.
>
> *—Eric (son 14 months)*

also be happy, excited, and fun to hang out with. If you're lucky enough to meet them (only with her permission, and never with a handshake), you'll discover they are unlike any breasts you've ever met before. They are bigger, more sensitive, and topped with a darker and larger areola (or nipple). And don't be alarmed by an extremely large nipple or two or three (well, three might be alarming).

Most women will go up a cup size (or more). This means a woman with small breasts will have medium to large breasts. Some men will be inspired by their partners' new pregnancy breasts.

A lot of men express a deep appreciation, curiosity, and fascination when it comes to their partners' new larger breasts. Whether you're a large breast man or just a large-breasted man, temper your excitement when you see your pregnant partner's breasts growing larger. A man who gets too excited is a man who risks getting into too much trouble. A man who falls over his partner's new big breasts (not literally, but possibly) might give the impression he's dissatisfied with her regular everyday breasts. Women are very sensitive to this and your appreciation can be misunderstood. What a woman doesn't realize is that the majority of men appreciate touching any kind of breast—be it small, medium, large, extra large, jumbo—we're just happy to be near one (or two). The excitement of bigger breasts isn't necessarily the

If he only knew that those great boobs I had would be tiny again, and no longer perky, he would have enjoyed them more...

—*Misti (daughter 2 years)*

PREGNANCY Q & A:

QUESTION: What should a man never do?
ANSWER: Mishandle her tender breasts.
(Suzanne, pregnant)
Focus too much on the boobs...they are huge, sore, and become really unsexy during pregnancy!
(Carin, mother of one)
Suck on her tender breast.
(Deb, mother of two)

QUESTION: What freaked out your man the most?
ANSWER: How giant my breasts were.
(Michele, mother of one)

size, but the experience of something different. It's the cherry on top.

Still, no matter how wonderful, exciting, and interesting you think her new breasts might be, don't let your appreciation get out of control. When you get the urge to say something about her size several times an hour, instead tell her how much you love her entire pregnant body. If you just want to talk about her new breasts, ask her what she thinks of them. If she tells you that she finds them terrific, feel free to agree. If she tells you that she finds them sore and always in the way, do not offer to massage them and get them out of the way (not sure what that means).

BREAST NOTE

If your partner is nursing (breastfeeding), her breasts will often be sore, tired, and not interested in your attention. Once your baby is done feeding, her breasts will need to rest. Should your partner invite you to hang out with her and her new breasts, be careful if she's nursing. Leakage, spraying, and dripping can occur. Safety goggles might ruin the moment, but be aware of the breast hazards.

THE BOTTOM LINE:
Ample, sizeable, immense, voluminous, enormous, gigantic, mammoth, mountainous, and titanic pregnancy breasts are for feeding the baby—not your sexual appetite. Look, but ask before touching.

Tip #34
THE VOMITING PREGNANT WOMAN: A Sense of Smell That Crime-Sniffing Police Dogs Envy

THE TIP:
Ask what she needs and avoid creating new odors.

THE STORY:
It was like having the flu without the temperature. It would hit me at night. I was throwing up about two to three times on a regular basis. We were living in a one-bedroom apartment so my husband was always close by, but he gave me my space. I didn't want him on top of me. He would always ask me what I needed. It had to be soup—chicken soup, matzo ball soup, or if it was late, wonton soup or some kind of broth-based soup. I

always had a metallic taste in my mouth and didn't like canned soup—it had to be homemade. My sense of smell was magnified a hundred times. Garbage odors and a combination of food smells were the worst. I would walk into a grocery store and want to vomit. I even had smelling hallucinations. When we moved into our new house, I was convinced that I smelled something dead in the kitchen. I'd ask everyone if they smelled it too. I would point to a place on the ground and they would literally get on their hands and knees to smell whatever it was that was bothering me. Everyone believed me, but no one smelled it. I think it was just a first-trimester thing. Eventually it went away.

—Lisa, son 20 months

✳ ✳ ✳

They call it morning sickness, but it can hit morning, noon, or night. Some women don't get sick at all. Other women get so sick that the vomiting can go on for months (but most will stop getting sick early in the second trimester).

It sucks to watch someone you love go through this gut-wrenching experience. It's a helpless feeling. And after a while, you start to worry about the kid getting tossed around when she

She was so sick, she was on anti-nausea medication—the same kind they give cancer patients—for five months.

—Kenny (twin daughters 2½ years)

176 • Dad's Pregnant Too

tosses her dinner. Don't worry. The baby will be fine. Once the nausea passes, it will fade from her memory, but while it's happening, there's not much you can do about it. Just ask her what you can do for her.

When and where it hits is unpredictable. It can be at home during breakfast, in the mall, at dinner, in the middle of an intimate moment in the bedroom, in the car, on a plane, on a train, on a bus, in an elevator, on an escalator, or on a moving walkway at the airport (I love those things). But typically, it's a smell that puts them over the edge.

Why does morning sickness happen? The cause is not completely known, but it's most often thought to be associated with a response to the surge of estrogen and other hormones as well as the relaxing of the stomach muscles, which means food empties more slowly. If it starts at all, it typically begins in the beginning of the first trimester and subsides in the beginning of the second trimester. But it can keep going well into the third trimester (women with multiples, first-time moms, and younger women can have more severe symptoms).

While you can't stop it, there are ways to help:

- Have some crackers or food nearby at all times. Eating something before bedtime and in the morning can help curb the nausea. Keep a little

I threw up most nights and couldn't sleep at the end of my first pregnancy. He held my hair and stayed up with me. But it didn't help when he told me that throwing up wasn't helping out the baby.

—Emily (son 21 months and daughter 3½ years)

Up to 70 percent of expectant moms experience nausea and vomiting

(Source: *Mayo Clinic Guide to a Healthy Pregnancy*)

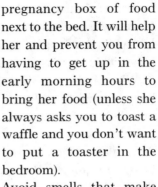

pregnancy box of food next to the bed. It will help her and prevent you from having to get up in the early morning hours to bring her food (unless she always asks you to toast a waffle and you don't want to put a toaster in the bedroom).

- Avoid smells that make her sick (lay off the heavy cologne).
- Don't get angry at her for being sick or tell her to suck it up (yes, this has happened). It's normal and it will pass.
- Encourage her to eat smaller and more frequent meals.
- Ginger ale and ginger candies (with real ginger) can help curb the nausea.
- Cook her less greasy foods and more bland foods (don't use the deep fryer).
- Make sure she gets enough rest (this might mean sending her to bed early).

- Talk to your care provider about acupuncture, antinausea bracelets, and prenatal vitamins (sometimes they can cause nausea). Also, ask your care provider for advice on when to seek help. Weight loss, vomiting blood or material that looks like ground coffee beans, and no signs of improvement require medical attention.

THE BOTTOM LINE:
Billions of women have vomited billions of times, and billions of these women have had healthy babies. Focus on taking care of her, and the baby will take care of itself.

Tip #35
THE FEELING FAT PREGNANT WOMAN: So Much More of Her to Love

THE TIP:
The more weight she gains, the more often she needs to be reminded of how beautiful she is.

THE STORY:
Unfortunately, I have gained more weight than I wanted to. So far I've gained 40 pounds. I was 130 pounds at 5' 8". I'm now 170 pounds, and I'm going to gain more. I don't think I'll hit 200 pounds. Getting

dressed in the morning is the worst experience; I never know what will fit me.

Some people feel really beautiful when they're pregnant. But I don't feel beautiful; I feel swollen, huge, and unattractive. When I look in the mirror, I recognize my body from the head up but from not from the head down.

The doctor says I'm totally fine. It's particularly hard because all my friends gained 25 pounds during their pregnancies. My husband is totally supportive and says that everyone's body is different. He knows it bothers me. It probably kills him to see me look in the mirror and get so upset. He's as physically attracted to me and maybe even more so. He tells me I'm more beautiful because I'm carrying his child— even more beautiful than I was before—and I tell him, "You're such a liar." But it helps to hear the words over and over again. There's no doubt that I'll get back to my weight.

—Allison, 7½ months pregnant

✳ ✳ ✳

This is one of the most sensitive and delicate issues.

So much of pregnancy is so uncomfortable. And to top it off, her expanding body is growing out of yet another pair of pants. A preg-

> If he thought I was too fat, he wouldn't bring me home cookies, right?
> *—Anonymous*

nant woman will have good days and bad days. A bad day

is when she grows out of her thin jeans. A good day is when a stranger flirts with her in the midst of a second-trimester "fat day" (don't be jealous, let her have it).

Some women find gaining weight liberating and others find it humiliating. Most women will gain 25 to 35 pounds (most guys about 10 pounds). Some gain more, some less. Avoid monitoring her weight. The end of her first trimester (possibly sooner) will be the end of her pants. The end of the second trimester will be the end of seeing her feet. The end of the third trimester will be the end of wearing clothes with a waistline. As her shape disappears, she needs to be reminded of the things she can't see—and that's our job.

As a partner of a woman gaining weight, my best advice is to make her feel beautiful. Some women love their new weight. They find it liberating to no longer have to worry about measuring up to the unattainable body image that society (and men) impose on them. Others feel fat, ugly, and disgusting. Whichever way she feels, compliment the hell out of her on a regular basis—this way, when she has a bad day and you tell her how beautiful she is, it won't look like you're making it up. She will believe you.

From the point when she grows out of her regular jeans until she has the baby and gets back into them (nine months up and at least nine

The first thing he bought me after I had the baby was a jogging stroller to help me lose weight. I told him it hurt my feelings because it made me think that he thought I was fat. He said he honestly knew I'd want to get back into shape and was buying it to please me.
—*Gini (daughter 4 months)*

months down), remind her of how beautiful she is. Find something beautiful to focus on. It can be her smile, eyes, belly, or her courage. If you can't find anything beautiful to compliment her about, then see a therapist. I'm completely serious about this. If you can't find anything beautiful about your pregnant partner, that's not something to ignore.

Following are some things you should *never* say or do and a few things you should *always* say and do:

- NEVER question how much she's eating (talk to the doctor if you're concerned).
- NEVER ask her if she really "needs" to eat something.
- NEVER ask her, "Are you sure you're hungry? You just ate."
- NEVER joke about how much she eats or the foods she eats.
- NEVER joke about her weight (even if she jokes at first, it will come back to haunt you).
- NEVER buy her clothing that's way too big (buy it with her or get a gift card).
- NEVER use the word *cellulite*.
- NEVER point out the areas where she has put on the most weight.
- NEVER tell her she's catching up to you.
- NEVER point out a problem without having a solution in mind.
- NEVER ask if everyone gains *this* much weight.
- NEVER compare her weight to other pregnant women's weight.

- ALWAYS tell her how beautiful she is.
- ALWAYS tell her how sexy she is.
- ALWAYS answer "No" when asked, "Do I look fat?" (she looks beautiful and pregnant).
- ALWAYS answer "Yes" when asked, "Do you like my body?"
- ALWAYS compliment body parts you love (not just her boobs).
- ALWAYS give her hugs and kisses.
- ALWAYS tell her she does *not* look pregnant from behind.
- ALWAYS ignore stretch marks.

If you're worried about her weight, go to the doctor's appointment with her and ask the doctor about it privately. If she has a history of eating disorders, make sure she mentions this to the caregiver. Hormones and dramatic change can bring up old emotions and past eating disorders. In addition to a caregiver, she might need to meet with a nutritionist or therapist to ensure she makes good choices.

As a rule, *never* discuss eating concerns while she's eating. If you think she's eating too much or making bad choices, be careful how and when you bring this up. You should know that a pregnant woman will gain 2 to 4 pounds per month during the first trimester and 3 to 4 pounds per month for the second and third trimesters (25 to 35 pounds total). She will need to consume roughly 300 additional calories a day. If you sense that she's gaining too much weight, talk to the

EXPECTANT FATHER TRIVIA:

QUESTION: What makes up the weight she gains?

ANSWER: Baby 6½ to 9 pounds, placenta 1½ pounds, amniotic fluid 2 pounds, breast enlargement 1 to 3 pounds, uterus enlargement 2 pounds, fat stores and muscle development 6 to 8 pounds, increased blood volume 3 to 4 pounds, increased fluid volume 2 to 3 pounds = Total 24 to 32½ pounds

(Source: *Mayo Clinic Guide to a Healthy Pregnancy*)

doctor first (this is why it helps to go to the appointments). Do not make food the focus; make it about her physical health and mental health. If you do end up talking to her about it, do *not* bring the subject up while she's eating or naked (both vulnerable times). Discussing it at the wrong time will turn you into an accidental asshole (see Tip #17). Doing it at the right time will make you appear like a loving and supportive husband. Another good tip is to be active as a couple. Plan walks and other low-impact activities. Attend a prenatal yoga class or get her a gift certificate. Change your workout routine to accommodate her.

THE BOTTOM LINE:

Enjoy her new bottom line, remind her that she's beautiful, and enjoy the new body—it's like being with someone else without the guilt.

Tip #36
THE FARTING PREGNANT WOMAN: Pregnant Women Get a Pass When Passing Gas

THE TIP:
Make sure the neighbors aren't within earshot.

THE STORY:
At the end of my pregnancy with twins I was so over it all. I remember leaving for a Dr.'s appointment, my last follow-up prior to the big day. We were walking (I was shuffling at this point) to the car in our garage, and I don't know what came over me, but I suddenly stopped and just stood there, letting out the biggest fart ever. The sound of it reverberated off the walls of the concrete in the underground garage. It was so powerful there was an echo that trailed it. My husband and I laughed until we cried, and then all of a sudden he noticed one of our neighbors had just gotten out of her car. She heard the whole thing, and was so mortified, that when she passed by us, she couldn't even look at us. Mind you, this is someone we spoke with quite often. I really think she wanted to run. When my husband walked by he said, "If you think it sounds bad, you should smell it."

—Angela, twin sons 24 months

✳ ✳ ✳

In the words of my pregnant wife, "I know nothing about this one."

This might come as a shock to you (and to the woman you love), but all women expel gas. I know—your partner has somehow made you think that she doesn't fart, but she does. And if she has never broken wind in front of you before, take cover—her ass is about to explode.

Many women will become constipated during pregnancy. Along with this constipation comes frequent gas. A lot of pregnant women will constantly break wind. Some of you are used to your partner's frequent flatulence. Others of you are in fart denial (thinking she never expels). Some guys don't mind the gas. Some hate it. Some find it a turn on (weird, dude).

Through my personal and professional research, I've discovered that pregnant partners might break wind in bed, in the car, on a train, on a plane, at dinner, at the movies, or on a long road trip. When a pregnant partner breaks wind, what can a man do? Should your pregnant partner get a free pass when passing gas? How to handle her gas can present a serious moral dilemma. It's a question loving and supportive men have struggled with for generations. Options include:

Her gas was beyond normal. It would wake me up at three in the morning. Not the sound, the smell.

—*Chase (sons 2½ years and 8 months)*

a. Retaliate with one of your own.

b. Humiliate her by shouting, "Someone needs medical attention!"

c. Be a hero and take the blame for the public stink bomb by saying, "Excuse me."

But here's what I've discovered: Whether it happens on the highway, at dinner, or in the midst of a sweet goodnight kiss, instead of attacking or fighting her gas, exercise kindness and compassion. After all, she can't help it.

At the same time, encourage kind, courteous, and responsible passing of gas. Understand that the the first incident of broken wind is just a "tester." The tester is a test to see if the wind has an offensive odor. Once the offensiveness of the scent has been established, courtesy should be extended to you and everyone else in range. She can open a window, light a match, or spray air freshener.

WHY SO GASSY, BABE?

The increased progesterone has a relaxing effect on the gastrointestinal tract. This can lead to constipation, which can lead to gas. A few ways to relieve or manage the gas include drinking more water, eating smaller, more frequent meals, exercising, and asking you to leave the room when she feels the urge coming (you have to leave because she's the pregnant one). Avoid surprising her with meals of cabbage, cauliflower, onion, brussels sprouts, or bean casseroles. These foods are like jet fuel for the colon of a pregnant partner.

Every time I think I feel the baby moving, I fart.
—*Kelli (mother of one, pregnant with #2)*

And never retaliate with a fart of your own. The reason retaliation is a poor choice is because pregnant women have a strong sense of smell. Retaliation can trigger nausea, which can trigger vomiting. And that's just not fair.

THE BOTTOM LINE:
Your pregnant partner may have bad gas. If she blames it on the dog and you don't have a dog, let it go. That's part of being a loving partner.

Tip #37
THE HEMORRHOIDAL LEAKY PREGNANT WOMAN:
Kind of Like a Leaky Faucet

THE TIP:
If you see something, tell her about it, but wait until the right time. A women who just gave birth doesn't want to hear, "By the way, you have an inch-wide hemorrhoid bubble hanging out of your ass."

THE STORY:
When she was pushing, a lot of stuff was happening down there. But I did notice something appearing in her anal area. It was a little smaller than a small raisin. I didn't say anything to her because I didn't know what it was at the time. The female anatomy is a great mystery. When she told me a couple weeks later that

she had some discomfort, I didn't connect the dots (no pun intended). She went to the doctor and was diagnosed with a hemorrhoid. When she told me I said, "Not surprising—let me tell you what happened...."

—*Michael, daughters 2, 5, and 7 years*

* * *

As much as they're going through, women do *not* want to repulse and repel us. Sometimes they will avoid telling us things that embarrass them or make them feel uncomfortable. Sometimes we'll avoid telling them if we see something embarrassing. But one thing a man needs to know: Pregnant women may leak blood, fluid, urine, mucus, milk, or something else that you've never seen, touched, or smelled before. Women don't volunteer this information because they want us to think they're beautiful and attractive.

AUTHOR'S NOTE:

My wife just got over a bad cough. Sometimes her cough would get so bad that she would pee in her pants. She told me that she went through three pairs of underwear in one day. I only share this to suggest a loving gift for your pregnant partner when running to the drugstore to get her cold remedies—nothing says I love you like a box of incontinence pads.

I asked the doctor, "What's the deal with feeling like I wet my pants?" He said it was normal. I went home and told my husband that wet pants were normal. I want him to understand what I'm going through.

—*Stacey (29 weeks pregnant)*

GETTING TO KNOW HER LEAKAGE:

- **THE MUCOUS PLUG**: Should you spot bloody (brownish or red-tinged) mucous discharge in the third trimester, this is probably the mucous plug (it's what blocks the cervix). Losing her mucous plug usually means her cervix is dilating (opening up) and effacing (becoming thinner and softer). Labor could start right away or may still be days away.

- **AMNIOTIC FLUID**: The term *water breaking* refers to the amniotic fluid leaking from the amniotic sac (also called *rupture of membranes*). When her water breaks, it can be a trickle or a gush (only about 10 percent

As the pregnancy progresses, things might leak. There's going to be the mucous plug (also known as bloody show). There might be blood from a hemorrhoid. There may be amniotic fluid (if the bag of water should break). There is also urine from incontinence. If nursing, breast milk might drip, spray, or spritz at unexpected times (*do* tell her if wet spots suddenly appear on the upper half of her shirt). During the actual labor and delivery, you might see something that she can't see—things you never wanted to see or thought you would see.

Should you encounter something like blood or a strange odor, or if you just see something out of the ordinary, say something to her about it. Do not keep it a secret. A woman needs to know.

Knowing how to tell her takes some finesse. Pregnant

women want to know that you think they are beautiful, especially when their bodies are out of control. When you see or smell something, wait a few minutes until the moment has passed (if it freaks you out, wait until you're back under control before explaining what happened). When sharing uncomfortable information, I find the best approach is to sandwich the comment between two compliments. This wasn't my original approach (someone shared this with me but I can't remember who). First you say what you love about her, then share what you've seen, smelled, touched, or tasted (yes, it can happen). Once you share it, top it off with something that will remind her that you love her and that you still think she's beautiful.

If you just can't say it, then pull the doctor aside or

of women's water will break naturally).

- **URINE**: Don't try to make her laugh or tickle her; she will literally pee in her pants. The pressure of the baby on the uterus can make it hard for her to hold urine.
- **VAGINAL DISCHARGE**: Women will normally have an increase in vaginal discharge during pregnancy— not something you probably want to hear or talk about. If you find that it's odorless or barely has a smell, that's normal. If it's greenish, yellowish, grey, thick, or strong/ foul smelling, let her know. This could mean an infection.

have someone close to her say it for you. But someone needs to say it.

THE BOTTOM LINE:
If you see something that she can't see…touch something that she can't reach…smell something that she can't smell…tell her.

Tip #38
THE SPOTTING CRAMPING PREGNANT WOMAN:
Normal Stuff That Might Scare Her (And You)

THE TIP:
She might bleed—don't panic if it happens, but get a hold of your doctor or get her to a hospital to make sure it's nothing.

THE STORY:
She started bleeding late into the pregnancy. She was scared when she told me. She called the doctor, and we were told to go straight to the emergency room. The ride took forever, but we didn't have to wait around. The doctor examined her right away. The placenta was tearing from the lining of the uterus, which was causing the bleeding. We were lucky that we moved so quickly; it could have been much worse. It was too soon to deliver the baby so she was put on bed rest.

Staying in bed kept her stable. She had the baby a month later, about four weeks early. The baby was small, but healthy. That was our scariest moment.

—Steven, son 3 months

* * *

At some point she's going to turn to you and tell you she's having some pain, bleeding, cramping, or discomfort. And that's going to be the moment your world stops for a long second—even though it's probably nothing to worry about.

For example, at 16 weeks pregnant, my wife started getting cramps that were so bad she had to sit on the floor at Target while shopping. The cramps stopped and returned a couple more times. She called the doctor, who told her to stay off her feet and monitor the cramping. The cramping was either due to a bladder infection or related to her ligaments stretching. Now, I didn't exactly curl up in the fetal position and bite my nails under a blanket of fear, but it was a little scary to think something *could* happen. And something worrisome will probably happen to you at some point. (But always contact your caregiver.) Assume it's nothing until it's something.

During our first pregnancy, at week 38 my wife had sixty minutes of contractions. They seemed like real labor as opposed to false labor (see the sidebar on p. 195), exhibiting all the symptoms of the real deal:

1. They occurred at regular intervals.

BLEEDING:

Up to 25 percent of pregnant women have light vaginal bleeding, or spotting, during the first trimester. In most cases, spotting (light bleeding) is not a sign of a problem. But always have her check with her caregiver.

(Source: *Mayo Clinic Guide to a Healthy Pregnancy*)

2. They lasted at least thirty seconds and got longer in duration.
3. They didn't go away when she changed positions.
4. They were in her lower back and lower abdomen.

I insisted that she was in labor and told her to start packing. I tracked each contraction in a notebook. After an hour, she got tired of counting and fell asleep. Three weeks later we had the baby (and no, she wasn't in labor for three weeks, they were just Braxton Hicks).

Part of being pregnant means experiencing aches, pains, discomfort, and possibly bleeding. Contractions and cramping will happen at some point. Call your caregiver if you're concerned. But make it a rule to call if she experiences the following symptoms:

- Bleeding or leaking fluid from the vagina
- Sudden or severe swelling in the face, hands, or fingers

- Severe or long-lasting headaches
- Discomfort, pain, or cramping in the lower abdomen
- Fever or chills
- Vomiting or persistent nausea
- Discomfort, pain, or burning with urination
- Problems seeing or blurred vision
- Dizziness
- Sensing a change in the baby's movement
- Suspecting the baby is moving less than it normally had been after 28 weeks of pregnancy (if you count fewer than ten movements in two hours or less)

FALSE CONTRACTIONS (BRAXTON HICKS): The uterus's "practice" contractions can start as early as week 22. One way to tell that they're practice contractions is to have her change her position (from sitting to lying down, or from sitting to walking). If the movement slows or stops the contractions, it's most likely false labor. Real contractions will continue and get more intense. Whatever the contractions end up to be, have her call your caregiver to make sure it's not preterm labor.

When something doesn't feel right, call your caregiver. Don't worry about being annoying. And a serious reminder: This book is *not* a medical guide. Your caregiver is your guide; always call your caregiver when you suspect a problem. If you want more information while waiting for your caregiver to return the call, check out the *Mayo Clinic Guide to a Healthy Pregnancy* or consult a website you trust for some clinical information. You can also check out MedlinePlus: www.nlm.nih.gov/medlineplus/. It includes a list of resources and publications from respected sources. But again, none of these are substitutes for talking to your doctor.

Just know that the contractions, cramping, and even bleeding can be normal. While you're waiting for the doctor to call you back, you can reassure her that this is the part no one tells you about.

THE BOTTOM LINE:
I never knew that bleeding and cramping were normal. I wish someone had told me.

Tip #39
THE NEVER-SO-TIRED PREGNANT WOMAN: Making Narcoleptics Look Well-Rested

THE TIP:
If a woman says she's tired, help her; don't criticize her.

THE STORY:
I was so exhausted from just being pregnant and he was supposed to help clean the house. I really needed to take a break. When I told him I was going to lie down, he said, "I don't know where, there's crap

everywhere!" I immediately felt guilty about lying down and forced myself to keep going. I remember being in tears because I was so tired, and my back hurt. He really didn't understand how tired I was. I should have been more vocal. The second pregnancy I started to speak up.

—Hannah, son 1 year, 5 weeks pregnant

✳ ✳ ✳

When I get sick and need attention, I tend to be dramatic. So I sometimes wonder if women who are pregnant act dramatic, knowing that being pregnant gives them license to be dramatic. There will be times when your partner says and does things that will make you question whether she's being entirely truthful or simply adding drama. When you sense some drama, the best advice is not to say anything about the suspected drama. In fact, I made this mistake so you don't have to. Here's what happened...

At the time my wife was 9 weeks into her second pregnancy. We had a conversation on the phone during which it sounded like she could hardly push the air through her lips to form words. I was having a busy day at work and didn't have the patience for her tired voice. It slowed me down and annoyed me. I couldn't imagine anyone being so tired. It struck me as a little dramatic. I should have just kept my mouth shut. I knew better. Yet for some reason I couldn't keep quiet.

Later that night I asked her, "Were you being dramatic or were you really that tired?" She asked me to repeat the question; she couldn't believe her ears. The question was *that* shocking.

She responded that she never felt so tired in her life and that she didn't appreciate me calling her dramatic. I explained that I didn't call her dramatic. I further explained that if she wasn't that tired, it could have been interpreted as dramatic. I wanted to understand how she was feeling so I could be a more under-standing partner. She told me that she couldn't believe I'd ask her such a stupid question. She didn't call me stupid, she called my question stupid. But her tone screamed, "You insensitive dumbass!" I felt bad that I hurt her feelings. And now I understood that she was *that* tired.

How a pregnant woman feels should never be ques-tioned. If you sense that she's being too dramatic, keep it to yourself. We are programmed with internal wiring that tells us not to say such things (my wiring failed). If you have the urge to question her level of drama, share it with me or share it with a stranger—better yet, tell your dog. (If you don't have one then get one so you have someone to tell.)

What I also learned is that this tired thing is for real. It starts in the first trimester and continues for the next eighteen months. The first trimester sucks all the energy out of some women. The second trimester makes sleeping uncomfortable. In the third trimester, she's restricted to sleeping on her side—assuming she sleeps at all. Running to the bathroom, getting kicked by the baby, and dealing with the issues described in Tip #34 and Tip #40 will give her reason to be completely, fall-on-her-face, never-so-tired-in-her-life exhausted.

If your partner is working while pregnant or taking care of other kids at home, she might have nothing left for you when she gets home. She'll need help with dinner, dishes, and the things she used to do (assuming she did these things). For guys who are used to sitting on their asses, this can be shocking. Just appreciate that every time you help her out it will make her feel that much less tired and that much more supported.

HELP HER, AND HELP YOURSELF:

As you'll read in Tip #57: Seducing Your Pregnant Partner, cleaning and helping around the house will help her save her energy for later. In the words of one woman, "She has a finite amount of energy. Helping out means she might be able to expend some energy on you."

THE BOTTOM LINE:

Ask a tired pregnant woman if she's being dramatic and you'll see true drama unfold.

Tip #40
THE SNORING RESTLESS PREGNANT WOMAN: Like Sleeping on the Tarmac of the Airport

THE TIP:
They should call the couch a bed because it's where you'll do some of your best sleeping.

THE STORY:
I've never been a good sleeper in a room with noise. My wife was a great silent sleeper, the secret to our marriage. She never snored until she got pregnant. Then she would constantly shift around. She would go to the bathroom several times a night. I didn't complain. I got up and slept on the couch because it was the only place I could sleep. We never talked about it. It was like my place was on the couch, and no one needed to talk about it. She didn't miss me. I enjoyed my couch.

—Gary, sons 2 years and 6 months

* * *

I'm a stomach sleeper and need to be a side sleeper. So, I bought a long pregnancy pillow so I don't roll over on my back. He uses it more than me.

—Stacey (25 weeks pregnant)

Sleeping in the same bed with a pregnant woman is like sleeping on an airplane in the middle seat on a packed

eight-hour flight overseas. It's a series of constant inter-
ruptions. You might get some sleep, but it's broken
sleep. And it's not like you can change your seat or get
mad at the person in the seat next to you. (You can, but
it will get you a seat on the couch either way.) You'll get
pushed out of bed. You'll get woken up to run errands.
You'll be woken up in general, but it's not her fault.

Here are some common issues pregnant women
have with sleeping:

- The expanding uterus puts pressure on the
  bladder. Constant pressure on the bladder can
  mean constant runs to the bathroom and
  constantly disrupted sleep (hopefully she will
  close the door).

- The growing baby will put pressure on the spine
  and the circulatory system. Therefore women
  can't sleep on their stomach or their backs late
  in the pregnancy. This can mean a lot of tossing
  and turning.

- Your sleeping partner will constantly be getting
  kicked and poked by the baby in the middle of
  the night. The moving baby can keep her up.

- Roughly a quarter of pregnant women will
  snore—these are the same women who didn't
  snore before they were pregnant (sleeping on her
  side and using breathing strips can help).

- Pregnant women get hungry at all times of the day
  and night. Sometimes she will wake up and need
  food. If she's too big or tired to get to the kitchen,
  you might need to get her some nourishment.

- Terrible leg cramps can keep her up at night—moaning and groaning (stretching, heat, and straightening the knee and flexing the foot can help).
- Pregnancy congestion may cause her to sneeze, snort, and blow her nose at all hours of the night.
- Heartburn, gas, constipation, aches, pains, general discomfort, anxiety, and hormones can make sleeping elusive for her and for you.

Any of these things might wake you up. If she wakes you up, never ever complain. Just go back to sleep or quietly move to the couch (unless moving to the couch would upset or insult your partner; in that situation, ask if she'd like you to quietly move to the couch).

THE BOTTOM LINE:
If she wakes you up, do not complain. Go back to sleep—unless she asks you to do something, then do it, and go back to sleep.

If you have something to add or feel a body type is missing, please send me a note so that I can include it in future editions. Send via www.DadsPregnant.com

6

THE MIND OF THE PREGNANT WOMAN

And the Expectant Mother Thong

Each woman's emotional experience with pregnancy is unique and unpredictable. Her mind is constantly racing. Each day can be filled with new emotions, concerns, and insights. However your partner's mind changes always remember this: If her mood swings and knocks you over, don't take it personally. Dust yourself off and trust that the swing will come to a rest—it just might take a few months.

Tip #41
THE HAPPY PREGNANT WOMAN: Enjoying the Perks of Pregnancy

THE TIP:
Some pregnancies can be smooth and easy. It's not at all as terrible or difficult as she thought it might be.

THE STORY:
My due date is tomorrow. I've had a really easy pregnancy the whole time. I feel lucky. I haven't had a lot to complain about. I think I've been even more relaxed while I'm pregnant as opposed to not pregnant. I've been learning to have perspective and appreciate how great life is. It's kind of a riot watching my body change. I love it. Every step of the way I didn't know what was happening. I was expecting to be bigger, but I wasn't. I was expecting to get sick, but I didn't. I was expecting to be more uncomfortable, but I wasn't. My husband and I just look at each other and shake our heads in disbelief because all we ever heard was how hard and difficult pregnancy is. We're surprised by how much we've enjoyed it. Do we know anyone who has had a smooth and easy pregnancy and didn't complain about

I was surprised at how many people didn't like being pregnant. I loved it. I couldn't figure out what was so awful about it. I felt cheated because my baby was born a month early.

—*Mandy (son 2 months)*

it? Not that I can think of. I feel like I'm an anomaly. It's been a breeze.

—Amy, 40 weeks pregnant

✳ ✳ ✳

Forget whipping out the empathy belly—some women love being pregnant. And for the women who don't love it, I would contend that some of those pregnant women will read this list of things to be happy about and realize pregnancy is the best thing that ever happened to them (or they'll burn this page). While you can't tell a pregnant woman that she needs to start being happy (for God's sake, never tell her to be happy), there's nothing wrong with reminding her of some of the perks, such as:

- Pregnant women must gain weight. In fact, it's her job. *Not* eating more and *not* gaining weight is a problem.
- People are nice to pregnant women. They hold doors open, give up their seats, let them cross the street first, and are less likely to be rude (minus the guy in seat 25D—see Tip #25).
- Pregnant women get positive attention. A husband, boyfriend, or partner will do whatever it takes to make her happy (at least most guys).
- Pregnant women get to do a lot of shopping. A lot of women love shopping. Turn to Chapter 9 and

get her excited (if she doesn't like to shop you can rip out those pages).

- Pregnant women can get better parking spots. Many busy malls reserve parking for pregnant and new moms. (There are no spots for new dads—now isn't that the most sexist thing ever?)
- Pregnant women get thick hair, glowing skin, and strong nails (usually).
- Pregnant women can be forgetful and people will understand. They can miss work, misplace things, and be foggy-minded, and no one will think anything other than the fact that they're pregnant.
- Pregnant women can pick the movies they want to see, eat where they want, and go home whenever they get tired.
- Pregnant women get large breasts without surgery. (This is something women with smaller breasts may enjoy.)
- Pregnant women get the entire bed to themselves (snoring, restlessness, gas, and constantly urinating tend to clear out a room).
- Pregnant women get gifts (jewelry, maternity clothes, massages, flowers, and other special treatments).
- Pregnant women have a place to rest their hands and somewhere to place snacks (M&Ms).
- Pregnant women create life—something men can't do. That alone is something a woman can take pleasure in.

THE BOTTOM LINE:
With so many perks to pregnancy, it's hard to imagine how a woman could complain…

Tip #42
THE HORMONAL PREGNANT WOMAN: Swinging on Her Moods Like a Monkey

THE TIP:
Hormonal pregnant woman (gunpowder) + clueless man (spark) = explosive situation.

THE STORY:
My wife told me she didn't like the taste of Morningstar Broccoli Cheddar Veggie Bites. I thought I was doing her a favor by trying to get them out of the house. I made them for my lunch thinking I was doing good because now she wouldn't have to see them in the freezer. I was all proud of myself when she walked into the kitchen. I had a big smile on my face and told her, "Good news, I decided to make the rest of the broccoli bites to get them out of the freezer!" She had a stunned look that turned into rage. She was *so* angry that I could be *so* inconsiderate to make these while she was in the house. The smell alone made her want to vomit. She already had a

When I would get very angry or cry, he didn't understand. I had to keep reminding him it was only hormonal.
—*Susan (son 4 years, 36 weeks pregnant)*

nauseating day, and this put her over the edge. She burst into tears and stormed away. I just stood there with my Morningstar Broccoli Cheddar Veggie Bites wondering what the hell just happened.

—Brad, son 2 years, 26 weeks pregnant

* * *

I would say that living with a pregnant woman is like walking on eggshells, but I can't say this for sure because I've never walked on eggshells. I tried walking on eggshells as part of the research for this book, but when I put eggshells on the kitchen floor, my pregnant wife got pissed because I got her clean floor dirty. So, while I've never actually walked on eggshells, I figured out that even if you try to walk on eggshells, you'll upset a pregnant woman. That's how sensitive things can be.

The flood of estrogen, progesterone, and other hormones coursing through her veins can make even the simplest conversations troublesome. For example, the other day my wife was telling me how ridiculously tired she was feeling. I said, "Sweetie, why don't you take a nap?" She replied, "I don't want to take a nap. I have things to do." I answered, "Then don't take a nap." She snapped back, "Don't tell me

The best thing to do is to be as mellow and helpful as possible. Also keep her out of situations in the third trimester where she is likely to take things out on unsuspecting waiters/beauticians/store clerks, etc.

—Jay (daughter 20 months)

what I can do! I know I don't need to take a nap." I was tempted to tell her, "Clearly, you're overtired and need a nap." But implying that she was crabby would only increase her level of crabbiness, and that's not going to make my life any better.

As a second-time expectant father, I know better. I know this wasn't really her—it was the hormones affecting her. Hormones are to blame for the road rage, the crying during Lifetime's *A Baby Story*, the lack of patience, and the general unpredictable nature of living with a pregnant woman. At least this has been my experience (not all women react this way). I genuinely feel bad for her that hormones cause her to say, do, and feel things over which she has little control. Sometimes she doesn't even realize why she's doing something. It's only after the hormonal haze passes that she finds clarity. She always gets her feet back on the ground and makes things better.

The hormonal pregnant woman tends to:
- Cry more often
- Cry more easily
- Become angry faster
- Become impatient quickly
- Lose (or misplace) her sense of humor
- Need and want more attention
- Be more critical of people around her
- Be more critical of herself
- Hide her feelings
- Feel confused and out of control
- Lash out at strangers (this can be fun to watch)

GETTING COMFORTABLE IN YOUR EXPECTANT THONG:

1. Accept that this will be naturally uncomfortable and unpredictable.
2. Look in the mirror and acknowledge the things hanging out of your thong that make you uncomfortable.
3. Find information, resources, and people who can help you get comfortable with the uncomfortable issues hanging out of your thong. Once you're comfortable with the uncomfortable, instead of overreacting, you'll be able to focus outward and be more supportive, compassionate, and empathetic.

Understand that the things you said and did before she got pregnant may affect her differently now. A joke that was once funny before pregnancy can become insulting and insensitive. A gentle touch can send her into a rage. A favorite move that you do in bed might get you kicked out of bed.

On top of the hormonal changes, another reason she might be extra sensitive is that as a first-time mom, she's likely to be uncomfortable in the Expectant Mother Thong. Let me explain: Throughout our lives, we fill different roles. Some of these roles are more uncomfortable than others. The more uncomfortable roles make us feel as if we're standing in front of a mirror wearing a tight thong (figuratively or literally). When you're uncomfortable in your thong, your worldview changes.

The littlest things can set you off. Innocent jokes are seen as insulting jabs. A benign comment isn't so benign. A friendly gesture can be seen as insensitive and mean.

Take the pregnant woman who is gaining weight—literally she's so uncomfortable in her thong (especially the pre-pregnancy thong that's four sizes too small). When she's this uncomfortable, any comment, look, or touch can be misinterpreted. That loving pat on her rear end can be interpreted as a signal that her butt is too big, when in reality you were just trying to be affectionate. The more uncomfortable she feels, the more likely she is to snap. Hormones just exacerbate these feelings.

But it's not just women. Expectant fathers aren't always comfortable in the Expectant Father Thong (sorry about the image). With all the changes we're facing,

THINGS THAT WILL SEND HER OVER THE EDGE:

1. Dismissing her feelings ("You're just hormonal, you'll get over it.")
2. Referring to her as moody, crabby, bitchy, etc.
3. Not listening to her and not acknowledging her feelings

THINGS THAT WILL BRING HER BACK FROM THE EDGE:

1. Regularly reminding her of how amazing and beautiful she is
2. Doing something out of the ordinary for her
3. Taking her out on a date (movie, dinner, coffee)
4. Listening and being there for her
5. Connecting her to professional help

it's hard not to take her reactions personally. But know that she's just uncomfortable and trying to find her way in a cloud of uncertainty amidst a hormonal haze. (**NOTE:** Everyone tends to be much more comfortable in their thongs the second time around—and that makes navigating through the pregnancy so much easier. But it takes walking through the unknown to get to this point.)

Should she freak out, cry, get angry, or have an irrational outburst, be forgiving and understand that it's not you. She's just trying to figure out what the hell is happening with her mind and body. It's just hard to not take some things personally when everyone is standing around in their thongs.

THE BOTTOM LINE:
When her moods swing, do your best to step aside and not take it personally. (This means working to get comfortable in your Expectant Father Thong.)

Tip #43
THE STRONG PREGNANT WOMAN: We Are Not the Superior Sex

THE TIP:
When you think she's being strong, tell her. Women like this.

THE STORY:

Throughout my pregnancy, my husband would tell me how strong I was and how much he appreciated what I was going through for us. I had a natural birth with no medication. He was there the whole time holding my hand through the contractions and the pushing. I didn't even realize it, but he later told me that I squeezed his hand so hard that it hurt him for days following the delivery. Seeing the pain on my face and feeling how tightly I squeezed his hand made him realize that he could never go through what I went through. He kept telling me this. Having him tell me this made me feel like he understood and that was a great feeling.

—Elena, daughters 5 years and 8 years

* * *

We are *not* the superior sex.

Let me explain: Men might act like they are stronger and better, but that's only because we know that women have superpowers. We might be able to lift more, but we can't create, nurture, and push life out of our loins—that's raw power.

What most men don't realize is that with advances in technology and medicine, we don't even need to exist. If women wanted to take over the world they could store our sperm and eliminate men. Considering we each have millions of sperm, women could inseminate themselves and create a world totally dominated by women. It's nice of women *not* to do this, but if we pissed them off enough, they could. The reality that women could be self-sufficient is probably one reason why men have tried to dominate and control women. It's threatening to know that we can be wiped out and the human race could still survive, even thrive, and smell good, too (women smell better).

The awesome physical and emotional strength of your partner might hit you during the ultrasound. It might sink in when you feel a kick in her belly. It might get you when she vomits twenty times in twenty days (and still works, makes dinner, and makes love to you). It might be during crowning (the top of the head coming out) or during the final push or during the baby's first cry. Where, when, and how it hits you can't be predicted, but at some point you will realize it. Women are emotionally and physically strong—it's awesome (and scary in a way), and they like to hear about it. It makes them feel good.

They like to hear that we can't do it. They like to know that we get it. It makes them feel appreciated and acknowledged. There's a good reason why men don't do the birthing in the family. Men can't even manage their emotions after a few drinks. Imagine a dude, totally sober, carrying twins at 32 weeks. He'd be beating up everyone so they could understand and feel his pain. That's why men don't get pregnant.

THE BOTTOM LINE:

We need to be nice to women or they will wipe us out and inseminate themselves for millions of years to come (cool idea for a movie).

Tip #44
THE CRANKY PREGNANT WOMAN: This Time, We Are Partly to Blame

THE TIP:

The most helpful thing you can do is not snap back even when she's at her worst. Instead tell her that you love her.

THE STORY:

After having two kids and having gone through this before, he knows where the crankiness is coming from and doesn't let it upset him. He knows that I get impatient, tired, sensitive, and exhausted. When I snap at him, he just lets it go most of the time. Once in a while he will tell me when I'm being a bitch, but generally, he doesn't fight with me. The other day, I sent him a snippy email, and he responded back to me, "I love you." Another time this week, I was helping him with some contract work (I'm an attorney, now full-time mom), and I called him up and started yelling at him that his secretary needs to proof his work because it wasn't professional. He just let it go. Even when I'm at my worst, he doesn't argue or fight.

> —*Bridgette, daughters 3 years and 1½ years,*
> *and 16 weeks pregnant*

* * *

The cranky pregnant woman is much different from the cranky not-pregnant woman. The big difference? If not for you getting her pregnant, she would just be cranky—not cranky *and* pregnant. The pregnant part means that her crankiness is directly related to you. This means that being cranky is not just her problem.

Some women will want you to be connected to their crankiness. This might manifest itself in wanting to make you cranky, taking the crankiness out on you, or just making you clean or do something that will take her mind off of her own crankiness.

Thankfully, there is a five-step plan to confronting her crankiness:

1. Focus your attention on her: Do not multitask; put the game on mute, hang up the phone, and give her your full attention.
2. Listen quietly, intently, and patiently: Make eye contact, but *never* roll your eyes or act like you're in a hurry.
3. Sympathize with her crankiness: Apply the nonforgiveness apology (see Tip #46).

4. Ask what you can do to help: Be genuine when asking and be willing to actually do something if she has a suggestion.
5. Stay out of her way: Give her space to be cranky (it will subside).

Let's look at how these steps would work in a real-life scenario. When my wife enters the room and gives off that cranky vibe, I will stop what I'm doing and focus my attention on her. When she speaks, I'll listen quietly, intently, and patiently (no interrupting or multitasking). If she explains that she's exhausted, I'll respond with, "I'm so sorry you're tired. That sucks." By acknowledging her crankiness, she knows that I'm aware of the problem. I also acknowledge that it sucks that she has to go through it and I don't have to go through it. Next, I will ask what I can do for her. Asking her what I can do accomplishes two things: (1) It means that I'm willing to make an effort to help, and (2) If she says "There's nothing you can do," it allows me the opportunity to watch TV, play video games, work out, or go online without becoming an accidental asshole. All that said, sometimes none of these things will help, but attempting to help is all we can be expected to do.

Should you find yourself in an argument with a cranky pregnant woman, winning isn't the goal. It's about ending the argument as quickly as possible. (Refer to Tip #46: The Irrational Pregnant Woman for how to diffuse the situation and give yourself permission to be wrong and still be right.) And whatever you do, never joke about her mood (at least not to her). Even if she finds it funny one day she might not find it funny the next (see Tip #42: The Hormonal Pregnant Woman). This includes *not* joking even if she jokes first. Her joke might be a trap; do not get caught in it.

If her crankiness and irritability don't stop, consider pointing your partner in the direction of a therapist or discussing her mood with her care provider. The crankiness and irritability can be symptomatic of a deeper issue like prepartum or postpartum depression (see Tip #49).

THE BOTTOM LINE:

Cranky pregnant women are different from cranky not-pregnant women. You got her into this, so attempt to make it better.

Tip #45
THE ANGRY PREGNANT WOMAN: It's Not about Us, It's about Them

THE TIP:

Some pregnant women are just angry and there's little we can do about it.

THE STORY:

During my first trimester, I was having a hard time with smells. He'd come home from work and cook dinner on our George Foreman grill—usually grilled chicken with vegetables and some type of noodles. Some nights he'd do it all himself. The smell of chicken on the grill nauseated me. Afterward, he didn't clean the grill right away so the smell would linger. I wouldn't tell him because I wanted to be angry. The testosterone levels got to me; it was easy to go from 0 to 60. It wasn't anyone's fault I was pissy, but I often just wanted to simmer in my anger. I wanted to feel bad for myself. I was going through all these changes during the first trimester and I wanted to feel like I was the only one who was ever pregnant—like me and my pregnancy were the only things going on in this world. I was focused on me. So, when the grill sat there, dirty and smelly, I wouldn't say a word. And then when he'd come home the next day, I'd clean it and tell him how angry I was about it.

—Effie, 39 weeks pregnant

* * *

If cranky is a simmer, angry is a boil.

If you've done nothing wrong, recognize that her lashing out at you could just be a product of her being uncomfortable, unhappy, and out of control. It could be her body, her mind, her identity, or other issues bubbling to the surface.

Given that she has so little control over her life during pregnancy, getting angry and watching you get angry might be one of the last things she can control. While allowing her to get you angry might mean giving her what she wants, there's only so much an expectant father should be expected to do in order to make her happy—being a verbal punching bag isn't one of them.

Now, if you've done something wrong (like leaving a dirty smelly grill sitting on the counter), and she has good reason to be angry, don't defend what you've done. Don't make excuses. That will just make her angrier. Admit your mistake. Wait until she cools down. If you insist on continuing to make her angry, this might be *you* exerting control over the situation because your life is so out of control. And that's just not a nice thing to do to your pregnant partner.

Assuming you're innocent, talk to her after she cools down. Ask what you can do to make her happy. If she's always angry, point her in the direction of professional care. Anger and irritability can be normal, but they can also be a symptom of deeper issues.

THE BOTTOM LINE:
Some pregnant women need an outlet for their anger. If she starts to beat up on you, get her a punching bag and step aside.

Tip #46
THE IRRATIONAL PREGNANT WOMAN: Letting Her Be Right Even If She's Wrong

THE TIP:
If you get yelled at for something irrational, give her time to realize she's wrong—she should come around.

THE STORY:
My wife was having a bad day and I wanted to help her out. I have honestly never done dishes before. I washed the plates and loaded everything in the dishwasher while she took a nap. When she woke up, she saw the way I had loaded the dishwasher and said, "I can't believe how obnoxiously you loaded the dishwasher." She thought I should have loaded it with more dishes before running the cycle. I thought she was lucky that I took the time to load the dishwasher. After bitching me out, she went back to whatever it was that she was doing. It took her about eight hours to realize that she was wrong. I didn't argue with her at the time. What's the point? When doing nice things for your wife, make sure you do them the right way. To this day we joke about the "obnoxious loading" of the dishwasher. I have yet to put dishes in the dishwasher since.

—*Jim, daughter 2 months, son 3¼ years*

✳ ✳ ✳

Arguing with a pregnant woman in the midst of an irrational outburst is like arguing with a drunk in the midst of dime beer night. There's no point in challenging someone in an altered state of consciousness. There's a time and a place to pick your battles, and during an irrational pregnant woman's outburst isn't one of them.

I started writing this book with fading memories of our first pregnancy. I'm now in the midst of the second trimester of our second pregnancy. While my wife is dealing with a lot of the same issues, this second time around is different for me. For the first time in my life, *I don't have to be right to be right*. What I mean is that I don't need her to tell me that I'm right to know I'm right. I'm not saying that I'm always right. In fact, I'm an expert at being wrong. But when she is wrong, I don't need her to see it my way and according to my timeline: *I can be right and wrong*.

Sometimes I'll even apologize for upsetting her even if she's wrong. I use the "nonforgiveness apology" to diffuse the situation. This form of apology acknowledges that she's upset and that you understand. You say, "I'm sorry if I upset you," and that's it. It's the same as her having an ache or pain and you saying, "I'm sorry you're so uncomfortable." You're not seeking forgiveness—just offering compassion.

Truly, when I'm right and she's wrong, I do feel bad for her. About 99 percent of the time, she apologizes later, once her head clears. If something really bothers me and

> You just can't win. So just don't try. Just be wrong and be happy about it.
> —Mark (sons 10 months and 2½ years)

she doesn't apologize, I'll revisit the issue at a different time and in a different location. Then I'll explain myself and leave it at that. Other times I'll just let it go because I know she's pregnant and dealing with a lot.

Now, I'm not saying you should always let things go (that's called being abused). It's important to talk about the big issues, but it's just as important to pick the right time and the right place to talk about them. As a first-time expectant father, you might think you have a right to be right. But all that does is make you wrong. Even if you're right and she's wrong, upsetting her when she's in a tired, exhausted, and overwhelmed pregnant state of mind can be viewed as wrong. Then, while you were right all along, you'll still be wrong.

THE BOTTOM LINE:
Sometimes being right means giving her permission to think you're wrong even when it's glaringly obvious that you're right.

Tip #47
THE SCARED PREGNANT WOMAN: You'd Be Scared Too If It Were in You

THE TIP:
Remind her of all the things she's doing right. Keep reassuring her that everything will be okay. She might need to hear it over and over again.

THE STORY:

The fear of the unknown was the worst. For a while, a part of me believed a C-section might be easier because I understand surgery and can relate to it. Having a C-section would mean not doing the pushing and going through labor. In retrospect, I know how much better it is to deliver vaginally. My recovery has been far easier than friends and family members who have had C-sections. One thing that helped me: When I told him that I was kind of scared, he would tell me that I was doing everything I could to prepare, and he would actually run down the list of all the things I had done right. He'd remind me that it was going to be okay. Hearing that I had done everything I could do to have a healthy pregnancy reassured me. The anxiety I felt before giving birth was far worse than the actual birth.

—Kate, son 2 weeks

✳ ✳ ✳

I left the prenatal class crying because I realized that although it was quite easy and fun for the baby to get in there, it wasn't going to be so much fun to get it out. My husband was very comforting and kept telling me that once I actually went into labor, the only thing I'd care about was getting that baby out, and he was right.

—Jenn (daughter 2 years)

While we were driving, my wife would sometimes say, "How can a baby come out of me?" She'd look at her stomach and say, "I like my stomach. I don't want to gain weight." Then she'd say, "I'm too young to be a mom." This would be normal if she were pregnant, but she wasn't pregnant. We weren't even trying.

And that's exactly the point, the being scared part starts years before you or your sperm enters the pregnancy picture. Until you've gone through pregnancy and childbirth, it's impossible to know what it will be like, and that's scary. That's what it means to fear the unknown.

She might be scared of the pain, labor and delivery, complications, miscarriage, finances, the doctor, caring for the baby, getting a C-section, pushing, being able to nurse, pooping while pushing (a common fear), the possibility that her body will turn you off (especially after pooping while pushing), what happens after the baby is born, your marriage, parenting issues, and everything else that will happen as you continue this journey into the unknown.

Here are some things you can do to calm her:

1. Remind her that being scared is normal. All these changes, the prospect of pain, the medical issues, and the responsibility are very scary. If she wasn't scared, something would be wrong.

2. If it were so terrible, women wouldn't keep having children. Everyone would have one and be done. Having a child connects her to all the women who have done it before her. Encourage her to connect with other moms who have

> She's not the first, and she won't be the last. That's what I told my wife when she got scared.
>
> —*Franco (father of one)*

been there and done it. That connection can help get her through this. She's not the first and won't be the last.

3. Encourage her to talk to her caregiver about her questions and fears. Suggest that she make a list (or you can make one) of the things that concern her. If she can't talk to her doctor, she needs a new doctor or a therapist.

4. Participate in the pregnancy with her—prenatal appointments, birthing classes, shopping, reading her books. Your participation will help her feel like she's not alone and that you're in it together.

5. Consider getting a doula (a doula is a birth coach who will help reassure her before, during, and after the birth). (See Tip #4.)

6. Listen to her and hold her. Just being there quietly will make her feel secure and safe. Silence can speak volumes.

For me, one of the hardest parts of seeing her so scared was that it scared me a little. But being scared is a normal part of the experience. It doesn't make anyone weak or wrong—only normal. And feeling it together means being even more deeply connected.

Once you can get comfortable with the uncomfortable and allow yourself to *not* always know what's going to happen, you can focus your energy on the things you can control. Being there for each other is one of the things you *can* control.

THE BOTTOM LINE:
If she's scared, help her see that billions of women have done this for millions of years—proof that this can't be all that bad.

Tip #48
THE NESTING PREGNANT WOMAN: Cleaning House with Your Toothbrush

THE TIP:
If she talks about hanging a large chandelier in the nursery, it's time to intervene.

THE STORY:
I was obsessed with the nursery. I would come home from work and do nothing but search websites, cut and paste pictures into a PowerPoint slide show, and design the baby's room. I picked out an over-the-top chandelier (we live in a condo with low ceilings), a beautiful antique-looking iron crib (that cost $40,000), and gorgeous bedding ($1,500+). My husband would come downstairs and watch me. He wasn't pushy; he let me do it for a while. I would sit in my pajamas, eat ice cream, and decorate this fantasy room for hours. The crazy part was that I knew I was having a boy but insisted on creating a girl's room. This went on for about five weeks. Then one day my husband left to

work out and run errands. When he came back five hours later, I was still online right where he left me. He looked me straight in the eyes and told me this had to stop. Now I laugh thinking about that moment. That's when it sunk in that I was obsessed with a girl's room and I wasn't even having a girl. I realized it was stupid and stopped.

—*Christine, son 3 years*

* * *

Your partner won't actually build a nest. (If she does build a nest with twigs and leaves in your home, point your partner in the direction of professional help.) Nesting refers to the primal urge to prepare the home for the arrival of the new baby. The feeling usually hits in the second trimester and continues until the baby comes home to the nest.

Nesting is as much about control as it is about cleaning and organizing. This control theme is a constant throughout pregnancy. Having so little control means exerting control over things she can impact (your home, you, etc.). The Internet has opened up a whole new outlet that allows women to spend hundreds of hours searching for the perfect nursery items (it's futuristic nesting).

Nesting for a man means doing the things you've put off for years—things you never actually believed you would do, but talked about doing. When the nesting hits, she will become a cleaning-and-organizing machine, and she'll enlist you. Not participating at the very moment she wants you to participate can be interpreted as not wanting to be involved in the life of your new child (a big leap, I know). And the nesting instinct can strike her at the worst times—in the midst of a playoff game, on a Saturday night, after work, during lovemaking, or during dinner. If you're around when the urge hits her but don't want to participate, it doesn't really matter. When you see your pregnant partner in her ninth month carrying a bookshelf up the stairs, you'll find the energy to help.

THE EMOTIONAL PURCHASE:

If your partner, as part of her nesting, is spending money you don't have, see Tip #61: The Emotional Purchase.

When it happens, she will start throwing away things (sometimes things that don't need to be thrown away or things you still want). She might start disinfecting and scrubbing with a toothbrush (yes, my wife). She will arrange and rearrange. She might paint or do a project while you're at work. (Tell her to avoid paints—the chemicals in some paints are bad for pregnant women to inhale.)

The best advice is to talk about this before it hits her (try starting the conversation in the first trimester.) Put together a plan so that when her nesting instinct kicks in, you can remind her of the plan. Include a timeline as part of the plan, and stick to the plan or do things ahead of schedule. Then, when the urge hits, instead of getting pulled into her nesting, you can remind her that you plan to do it according to the timeline. But then again, she might say, "Screw your timeline" (that's some mouth on her) and grab the bookshelf. There might be no stopping her.

THE BOTTOM LINE:
Start nesting before she starts nesting by putting together a timeline—then you can nest on your own time (great in theory).

Tip #49
THE DEPRESSED PREGNANT WOMAN: The Most Important Tip in This Book

THE TIP:
If a guy sees his partner not playing with the kids or interacting, not getting out of bed, and not being herself, *he needs to get her help.*

THE STORY:

My doctor gave my husband and my mom her card. She told them to call if they thought I needed help. Carrying twins meant I was at greater risk. When the twins were first born, I was happy and excited in the hospital. They were healthy preemies. We left the hospital without both of them and that was very difficult. Once my first baby came home, I was tired, but I wasn't sad or depressed. Once the second came home, that's when the depression hit me. They were so needy and I had no time for myself. I'd wake up, feed them, feed myself, and pump (I never produced enough milk for a full bottle). Somewhere in between, I'd brush my teeth and get dressed. After I fed them, I wasn't that interested in playing with them or tickling them. It was like being in school and having to go to class. Every time they would wake up, I would go to feed them—I didn't want to, but I had to. They took forever to eat because they were premature, and feeding is so slow. They also had terrible reflux and cried for hours on end.

I didn't talk to my friends about these feelings because I didn't want them to know. I wasn't ashamed; I just didn't want them to think that I had mental problems. None of my friends told me they went through postpartum depression, and they couldn't relate to having twins. My husband was so helpful, but he was very worried about their health as preemies. Inside I was thinking, "I feel like crap and he's worried about their health."

When I went to the doctor for my six-week checkup, I told her what was happening and that I went to Target to do some shopping and didn't want to come home. She said, "You're the eleventh case of someone not wanting to come home from Target." The doctor prescribed some medication, and about three weeks later things began to get better. I started to want to interact more and be there for my girls. It's still hard for me at times, but I'm grateful I was able to get help and never endangered myself or my girls.

—Anne, twin daughters 20 months

✳ ✳ ✳

Postpartum depression (post-pregnancy) and perinatal depression (during pregnancy) need to be on your radar. According to the National Institutes of Health, postpartum depression (PPD) affects 10 to 15 percent of women any time from a month to a year after childbirth. What makes it so frightening is that it can happen to anyone reading this (10 percent of men suffer from postpartum depression too).

What makes it even scarier is that once you go back to work, you might not be around. You don't know what's happening at home and how she's feeling. She might be in pain and never tell you. She might have thoughts of hurting herself or

> Try and get a psychologist involved as soon as possible. When she doesn't want to get involved with her children, that's a sign she needs help.
> *—Steve (father of two girls)*

hurting the baby and keep them a secret. The good news is that treatment is available (medical and nonmedical), but she needs to get help in order to get better. And that means you need to be involved.

If you work long hours, travel a lot, or aren't around for hours at a time following the birth (up to a year) and you sense a problem, have your mom, mother-in-law, family, or her friends stop in and visit to make sure she's okay. If she exhibits any of the symptoms listed in this section or you feel that something isn't right, talk to her caregiver and get the name of a mental health professional.

A lot of women suffering from PPD will *not* seek help. She will call the doctor when she gets a cramp, but when the symptoms of depression surface, she'll keep it a secret. If at any point your partner exhibits any of the following symptoms (during or after pregnancy), and the symptoms last longer than two weeks, make sure you let her caregiver know. Here are some signs to watch for:

- Feeling restless or irritable
- Feeling sad, hopeless, and overwhelmed
- Crying a lot
- Having no energy or motivation
- Eating too little or too much
- Sleeping too little or too much
- Trouble focusing, remembering, or making decisions
- Feeling worthless and guilty

PERINATAL DEPRESSION:

Perinatal depression (depression during pregnancy) is so hard to diagnose because so many of the symptoms associated with it are a normal part of pregnancy. Again, this where having a relationship with your partner's caregiver and attending appointments can be so helpful.

- Loss of interest or pleasure in activities she used to enjoy
- Withdrawal from friends and family
- Having headaches, chest pains, heart palpitations (fast heartbeats or skipping heartbeats), or hyperventilation (fast and shallow breathing)
- Not interacting with or showing interest in the baby
- Fear of being alone with the baby
- Expressing thoughts of hurting herself or the baby

A FEW THINGS THAT EVERY EXPECTANT FATHER SHOULD DO

1. Bring up the risk of perinatal and postpartum depression early into the pregnancy. By helping your partner see that this is an illness that is *not* a reflection on how much she loves you or the baby, you help alleviate the shame. Treatment is available (medical and nonmedical). Men need to be

good listeners because if you don't hear her cries for help, you might miss her calling out for attention.

2. Sporadically check in with her during pregnancy and ask how she's feeling (you'll notice the doctor will do this if you go to appointments with her). It's way too easy to dismiss her moods and actions as hormonal. In reality, there could be more happening. If she's having a hard time, suggest she find a therapist she can talk to. Then once the baby is born, she will have built a relationship with someone she trusts. If you have to leave her at home alone, make sure people will be checking in and dropping by to visit.

3. Once the baby is born, encourage your partner to:

BABY BLUES OR DEPRESSION?

The baby blues can happen in the days right after childbirth and normally go away within a few days to a week. A new mother can experience sudden mood swings, sadness, crying spells, loss of appetite, and sleeping problems, and feel irritable, restless, anxious, and lonely. Symptoms are not severe and treatment isn't needed. Symptoms that linger more than a few days need to be discussed with your physician.

POSTPARTUM PSYCHOSIS:

In extremely rare cases—less than 1 percent of new mothers—women may develop something called postpartum psychosis. It usually occurs within the first few weeks after delivery. Symptoms may include refusing to eat, frantic energy, sleep disturbance, paranoia, and irrational thoughts. Women with postpartum psychosis usually need to be hospitalized.

(Source: The National Institutes of Health)

- Try to get rest—nap when the baby naps.
- Stop putting pressure on herself to do everything. She should only do as much as she can and leave the rest!
- Ask for your help with household chores and nighttime feedings. Ask you to bring the baby to her for feeding. Have a friend, family member, or professional support person help you in the home for part of the day.
- Talk to your family and friends about how she is feeling.
- Avoid spending a lot of time alone. Spend it with other moms, friends, and family.
- Spend time alone with you.
- Talk with other mothers, so she can learn from their experiences.

- Join a support group for women with depression if she thinks she may have PPD.

FOR MEN WHO HAVE PARTNERS SUFFERING FROM PPD

Being a partner of a depressed spouse or significant other can be overwhelming. You have to take care of her, the baby, and yourself. As important as it is for her to get help, it's equally important for you to find a support network. Find a group or one-on-one therapy. Essentially, you become a single father caring for the baby and your partner. There are several groups and websites for men with partners who have PPD. Care may also be covered under insurance.

THE BOTTOM LINE:

This can have a *happy* ending. Help in the form of nonmedical talk therapy and/or medication *are* available. And most people *can* be successfully treated. She just might need your help reaching out. And if it's you that needs support, don't be afraid to seek it out.

If you have something to add or feel a mind type is missing, please send me a note so that I can include it in future editions. Send via www.DadsPregnant.com

7

SPOILING YOUR PREGNANT PARTNER

Helping Her Feel as Good as She Feels Big

Tip #50
DATING A PREGNANT WOMAN: This Would Be Your Partner

THE TIP:

Your date doesn't have to be expensive or fancy. Making the effort will let her know you think she's still hot.

THE STORY:

I was *not* excited about leaving the house late in my pregnancy for a big Saturday night on the town. Besides getting tired at 8:00 p.m., I felt big and disgusting. My clothes felt like a tent. I also didn't like spending money. One night in particular, he surprised me and told me to get dressed up. I fought it the whole way. We got in the car and arrived at an inexpensive neighborhood Italian restaurant. He kept telling me how hot and beautiful I looked. I have no idea to this day if he was just saying it, but I didn't stop him. After dinner we saw a movie—the last one we saw for another nine months. What made it so special was that he made the effort, it was like he was still attracted to me and wanted to be with me. Yes, he did have a couple of drinks but only because I gave him clearance. Let me tell you, he earned those drinks—I wasn't the easiest preggo.

—Ally, daughter 11 months

* * *

You're probably thinking that you don't want to take on the added expense of putting your profile back on eHarmony, Match.com, or Jdate.com. But this tip isn't about dating other new people—it's about dating your pregnant partner.

When taking her out for a date, don't you dare even glance at that pretty thing on the other side of the room—especially after the baby is born when your wife really feels fat.

—Cathy (sons 4 months and 3½ years)

What's nice is that you've already met her (and gotten her pregnant), so asking her out on a date shouldn't be so intimidating (although she might have an early curfew). Given that she's pregnant, you know that she's not a virgin (so you might get lucky). One more bonus, she looks kind of different from when you met her. So, in a way, it's like dating a whole new woman. It makes for an exciting night on the town.

Once the kids drop into your world, things will be dramatically different (yes, everyone tells you this). But life will actually change for the better (few tell you this). That said, spending time together and doing things as a couple will take much more effort and planning once you have a child. In a few months, going out will mean finding a baby-sitter, paying for that baby-sitter, and pumping milk so that the baby-sitter can feed the baby if your partner is breastfeeding. (You don't actually have to pump them unless she asks.) Seeing a movie will cost you the price of the tickets, an additional $10 to $12 an hour (that's what people in Chicago pay for a sitter), plus popcorn, candy, and water.

Enjoy going out while it's easy, spontaneous, and cheap. You might be better off at a Saturday matinee and then grabbing dinner.

Besides taking advantage of this window of opportunity to have fun together, making the effort demonstrates that you still love her and want to be around her. Some women get paranoid that you will take off to the

When going out with a pregnant woman, respect her energy level and mood. If she doesn't want to be there, get out of Dodge. Make sure people aren't smoking nearby. She will be extremely sensitive to anything that might harm the baby.

—Mike (son 3 months)

RULES FOR TAKING HER OUT:

Make sure she can physically fit wherever you are going.

Make sure you don't accidentally walk too fast and leave her behind.

Make sure there are bathrooms, food, and drink nearby.

Make sure you can leave at any time if she gets really tired or emotional.

—Maggie, daughter 20 months, son 3 months

store for milk and bread and never come home. Spending quality time together goes a long way toward focusing on your life as a couple. And just like when you were single, if you want to have sex, wining (not whining) and dining her can increase your chances (as long as you get home before 9:00 p.m.).

Take her to dinner. Take her to a movie. Take her to a museum for the day. Take her to a sporting event (avoid making her walk to the upper deck). Take her to a concert (after week 26 the baby can hear the music too). Take her shopping for clothes. Take her to a spa for the day or night. Take her on a hike. Take her on a bike. Take her to an open mic (sorry for the rhyming sequence). Take her to another room in the house for a candlelight dinner you prepared (I mean, ordered in).

Take charge and give her attention. The goal isn't to get some action (although it improves your chances).

The goal is to connect as a couple; to remind her that she's beautiful; to shower her with attention; to remind her that she's loved; to help her laugh, relax, and have fun.

THE BOTTOM LINE:
Dating isn't about getting lucky—it's about showing her that you still care and love her. And, well, it's also about trying to get lucky.

Tip #51
THE BABYMOON: Getaway While You Can Get Away

THE TIP:
Go to a place where there are things to see—not people you need to see. Keep the travel time under two hours. Check with the doctor if your wife plans to have a glass of wine with dinner.

THE STORY:
We researched places to go and picked Washington D.C. Some of the warmer spots were too far to fly to, and at 32 weeks pregnant, she didn't want to sit for too long. We flew into D.C. around midday. We ate at a place called Old Capitol Grill, right next to the Capitol—I highly recommend it. Her doctor said an occasional glass of wine was fine, so she looked at the menu and ordered the most expensive glass. She said,

"If I'm going to have one glass, I'll have a good one."
She didn't finish it—I did. We toured the Capitol, the
Smithsonian, and a spy museum.

The trip was a last chance to spend an isolated
weekend—just the two of us. We didn't know anyone
there and that was a nice thing. If we had traveled to a
place where we knew friends or family, we might have
felt an obligation to meet up with them. It was great
because we don't know when the next vacation will be
together—and it won't be just the two of us! Right now
we're loving the experience of having our son in our
lives and seeing all the changes.

—Chris, son 2 weeks

NOTE: Check with your caregiver to see if wine is on
the menu. Ours said a few sips isn't a problem later in
the pregnancy, but that's a personal judgment call.

✳ ✳ ✳

Once you have your new baby, life will be different. (I
know you know this and are so tired of hearing this.)

Traveling and leaving home on a whim won't be as
easy. It will either mean taking your baby with you or leaving him at home. If she's nursing, leaving the baby at home means pumping milk for a few days beforehand. If

We planned a trip to Laguna Beach, California, in the second trimester. We went swimming, ate, walked around town—nothing too strenuous. It was perfect.

—Mandy (daughter 2 months)

you take the baby with you, this means bringing an infant seat, a stroller, a crib or Pack 'n Play, formula, bottles, sleepers, a monitor, diapers, diaper cream, bath soap, a baby bathtub, toys, burp cloths, blankets, and a bunch of other stuff I'm sure I missed. It also means working a vacation around nap times, bedtime, and 3:00 a.m. feedings. The baby is the center of attention.

The point of the prebirth vacation is that you as a couple are the center of attention. So, even if you're on a tight budget, it would be nice to find a way to get away and spend some quality time together as a couple (not a threesome). Pick a night or two or three to get away. If you're on a budget, keep it local and drive to a bed and breakfast a couple hours from home. If you have a bigger budget, avoid planning a surprise safari to Kenya. That's too long to sit on an airplane and she should be able to drink the water at your destination. Make it short and sweet. You might even opt for a package designed for pregnant couples (see the sidebar on the next page). If you do it right, the package will include a massage for two—which means you'll have to get one too.

If planning a prebaby vacation, the best time is early into the second trimester (the honeymoon period of the pregnancy). Make sure it's a refundable trip or buy travel insurance just in case (check if pregnancy is insurable). Other things to keep in mind:

- Keep the travel time less than a few hours. Sitting can be uncomfortable and may turn her mood south (even when driving east, west, or north).

THE CLIFFS RESORT'S "AND BABY MAKES THREE" PACKAGE FOR PARENTS-TO-BE:

Couples can enjoy their last romantic getaway as a twosome at The Cliffs Resort in California before baby makes three. This escape package includes:

- Welcome basket with diapers and a onesie
- Doc Burnstein's Baby Brickle ice cream
- Commemorative bottle of wine
- Two one-hour massages

- If traveling by air late into the pregnancy (within a couple weeks of the due date), a doctor's letter might be required to board the plane.
- Always check with your care provider before making any travel plans.
- If driving, make sure the seatbelt never goes over her belly—always low across her pelvic bone. Plan for a lot of stopping and anticipate pregnancy gas (see Tip #36).
- If going on a cruise, check the rules and regulations. Some cruise lines don't allow pregnant women beyond their 26th week on board. Bring a letter from the doctor just in case. Avoid first-trimester sailing—motion sickness plus morning sickness makes for a messy cabin.

- If traveling out of the country, check your health insurance plan to see if you're covered. If not, buy more insurance or change your destination.
- No drinking water at exotic ports of call outside the United States.
- If sitting for several hours, encourage her to walk around. Leg cramps, leg pain, and blood clots are possible complications.
- Consider getting travel insurance just in case she doesn't feel well enough to go (pregnant women can be unpredictable).

- $50 dinner voucher at the Sea Cliffs Restaurant
- In-room movie
- Breakfast in bed

Suggested website:
www.babymoonfinder.com

THE BOTTOM LINE:

A prebaby vacation can be the perfect getaway. Once you have the baby, it will be hard to get away.

Tip #52
THE PRENATAL RUBDOWN: Massaging Whatever She'll Let You Touch

THE TIP:

When giving her a pedicure, remember the base coat.

THE STORY:

I was on bed rest for several weeks, and my husband wanted to give me a pedicure. So, he bought loofa scrubs, lotions, and a foot tub; I already had all the polishes and picked out bright red—a really hard color to use. I think he put on a football game while he did it; I like it so I didn't mind. He did what he thought a full pedicure would be. He started by putting my feet in a tub. Then he scrubbed my feet and massaged them for five minutes. He didn't do any of the clipping. I preferred that he not do that. Then he polished my toenails. He didn't apply a base coat, and I got one coat of red. I didn't say anything to him—I said "Thank you!" I've probably had worse, but I wouldn't be a repeat customer.

—Renee, daughter 2 months

✳ ✳ ✳

Women like to be touched. Men like to touch women. (That's what got you into this situation.)

There are a lot of reasons to bring out the pregnancy massage, but the biggest reason is that it will help her feel better. It's proven to improve circulation and the elasticity of the skin; decrease swelling, muscle fatigue, and stress, and help with sleeping. And touching can lead to other things.

If you've never given a massage, surprise her. It can be a two-minute massage (and no, that's not slang for anything) or a twenty-minute one. Anything you can do is enough. The results will be dramatic. Besides connecting with her and possibly leading to action (see Chapter 8), it's just a nice to thing to do for her.

If you have never given a massage and don't want to give one, then get her a gift certificate for a massage at a spa, health club, or hotel. See if they have a certified prenatal massage therapist on staff; certain pressure points of the body have been thought to trigger

PREGNANCY Q & A:

QUESTION: What can a man do to increase his chances of having sex?
ANSWER: Massage the mom's feet/shoulders. Run a bubble bath for her (not too hot). Tell her she looks amazing and sexy (but only if you're being honest—she'll know if you're insincere). (Susan, pregnant, mother of one)

QUESTION: The perfect gift for a pregnant woman?
ANSWER: A gift certificate for a pregnancy massage. (Brittany, pregnant with #1)

Encourage relatives or friends to buy her a massage gift certificate. You can also get her one for Valentine's Day, Mother's Day, or some special day that you make up to celebrate her.

contractions. (Now, if you're in week 42 and want to get this kid out, have the massage therapist touch all the right pressure points. Hell, have the therapist show you.)

If you want to give a massage and don't know how to give one or are afraid of hurting her, schedule a massage lesson. You can do it as a couple. My wife and I took a couples massage class before she got pregnant (and it enabled me to get her pregnant). We learned techniques such as effleurage (long strokes from the neck to lower back using the whole hand), petrissage (a rolling and squeezing action using the thumbs and fingers), and friction (moving the thumbs and fingers in little circles to penetrate the muscle).

If you wing it, proceed with light pressure and avoid the ankles until your due date; certain pressure points can cause premature labor. The best position is to have her sitting down or lying on her side (not on her stomach or back). If you want to get serious about this and make it an activity, turn down the lights, create some mood music, bring out the massage oils, some candles, pillows, and towels, and go to town. The risk is that she enjoys it too much. Then she'll be expecting it all the time. But that's why there are gift certificates.

THE BOTTOM LINE:
Don't give a massage just to get some. Do it to help her relax.

Tip #53
MATERNITY CLOTHES: The Better She Feels, the Better Life Will Be

THE TIP:
Encourage her to buy maternity clothes. Buying bigger non-maternity clothes to save money is a bad idea that will cost you in many other ways.

THE STORY:
When I was pregnant the first time, my husband thought it would be a good idea to buy larger-size clothes instead of maternity clothes, which are only worn for nine months. The problem with bigger clothes is that they're not form fitting; they just made me look like a gigantic cow. He would go to the discount rack and pick out something in a size 14 for

me—I'm a size 6. We both thought it was silly to spend money on maternity clothes, but it's not a good feeling to feel ugly for nine months. During my second pregnancy, I splurged on maternity clothes. (When I say splurged, I mean shopping the sale at Gap Maternity.) I was so much happier. I felt pretty. I wanted to be more social because I looked nice. I was happier to go out and be with my friends. I felt less self-conscious. I looked cute. Because I was so much happier, it made being with me much easier. I wasn't nearly as crabby as I was with the first. The value of looking good and feeling good far exceeds the price, even if you will only wear it for nine months.

—Irene, daughters 7 years and 5 years, son 6 months

✳ ✳ ✳

You might be thinking that she's only going to wear these clothes for nine months, but it's the best money you can spend.

How she feels about herself will determine how she feels during this pregnancy. As her body changes, having something that looks good on can help make her feel more comfortable. If she thinks she looks like hell, those around her will feel the heat. If she enjoys shopping, great. If she's not a shopper, encourage her to get at least a few new things. (I know this seems self-destructive and

I *forced* her to let me spend a few hundred bucks on her. For some reason, she was the one resisting.
—Todd (son 4 months)

dangerous, but it will make life better for you and the rest of the world.)

When you find out she's pregnant or when she grows out of her pre-pregnancy jeans, get her a gift card to a maternity store—either a neighborhood boutique or a larger chain (she can shop online—see the sidebar on the next page). If you're going the boutique route, ask a friend of hers who has been through it for advice on where to go (and tell her to keep it a secret).

Warning: Some maternity clothes can be offensively expensive. I went shopping with my wife the other day and was blown away by the price of the jeans. I saw denim jeans for $275; I also saw some on sale for $25. Grudgingly, I admit that there is a definite difference. So when buying your gift card, walk around the store or check it out online and decide what you can afford to put on the card. Different stores have different price points. A saleswoman at one of the higher-end stores told me that the only fight she witnessed was between a husband and wife over a pair of jeans—he felt the jeans were too expensive; she didn't. One way to look at it is to amortize the jeans over a hundred days of wearing— $200 jeans would cost about $2 a day. Is $2 a day worth it to keep a pregnant woman happy? Sure (vigorously nodding my head so hard I think I pulled vertebrae).

If you're someone who likes to shop and thinks a gift card is impersonal, think again. Getting the wrong size—a wrong size that's way too big—can turn you into an

I know the jeans were ridiculous, but if it takes $200 to make my butt look cute when I'm pregnant, then so be it.
—*Tami (daughter 22 months)*

SPECIALTY MATERNITY STORES (BUY A GIFT CARD):

- Gap Maternity (www.gap.com)
- Old Navy Maternity (www.oldnavy.com)
- Ann Taylor Loft Maternity (www.anntaylorloft.com)
- Mimi Maternity (www.mimimaternity.com)
- Motherhood Maternity (www.motherhood.com)
- A Pea in the Pod (www.apeainthepod.com)

accidental asshole. Women don't like getting clothes ten sizes too big from the only man (other than the doctor, resident, and twenty interns) who sees her naked. Go with the gift card.

ESSENTIAL SHOPPING INFORMATION

- If you're shopping together as a couple, be careful not to be too blunt when hanging out near the dressing room. Never tell her she looks fat—tell her it's not the most flattering thing you've seen her wear.
- Maternity clothing has such a short life span that return policies are often restrictive (at boutiques or department stores). *Make sure she knows the return policy before buying.* Some women like to buy clothes, take them home, try them on, and then return them (I don't know any guys who do this).

- Encourage her to ask friends or family if they can share some of their maternity clothing. Most of the time, people are eager to share.
- When it comes to buying her maternity lingerie or clothing meant to make her feel sexy, shop with her or opt for the gift card. While you might have loving intentions, getting a piece of lingerie that's too big is a big-time rookie mistake.
- If she does buy a lot of high-end clothing, she can sell the items on eBay when she's done. Auctions can get pretty intense for maternity jeans.

THE BOTTOM LINE:
She needs to feel pretty or things will get ugly.

Tip #54
THE PUSH/PREGNANCY PRESENT: A Little Something to Ease Her Pain

THE TIP:
It doesn't have to be diamonds…

THE STORY:
The day I turned 20 weeks pregnant I got home after a *long* day and found a package and card on the table with "mommy" written on it. It was a card from my hubby and baby celebrating the fact that we are

halfway through the pregnancy. The present was a wooden Willow Tree figurine called "Cherish," which is a pregnant mommy holding her tummy. Then, yesterday, out of nowhere, Daddy and baby sent me a cookie bouquet (my *favorite*!)—six beautiful cookies celebrating that "It's a girl!" One of the cookies had Elizabeth's nickname on it, *Ellie*. I pretty much have the most amazing husband ever!

—*Valerie, daughter 1 month*

* * *

A Push Present is a gift given to your partner following the birth. The idea of buying a new mom a special gift once she pushes the baby out isn't just made up by her. It has roots. In Europe, it's customary for women to get a gift following the birth of a child. In England, men are expected to adorn women with a beautiful ring. In India, mothers get gold and jewels for the birth. In the United States, jewelers and women who want jewelry are turning this into a new gift-giving tradition.

Some guys aren't into the idea of a push present. It's

If *only* my man had known how painful it is to push a baby out of your vagina! He may have given me a push present!

—*Carin (mother of one)*

I got a "pushing present"/thirtieth birthday gift. I helped pick it out—a beautiful diamond necklace.

—*Heidi (mother of one, pregnant with #2)*

The best gift a man can get his wife? SLEEP!!!

—*Misti (daughter 2 years)*

not that these guys are cheap (although some might be). They say there is no greater gift than the gift of having a healthy new child, and a material thing like jewelry almost minimizes the magnitude of the event. The baby is the ultimate "push present." So, if you share this sentiment, there's nothing wrong with calling the gift something else. How about just calling it her first Mother's Day present and picking it out after the baby is born? Call it a gift from the baby and make the baby pay you back when she's old enough to work. Whatever you subscribe to, I have a hard time finding anything wrong with getting someone you love a gift that's associated with such a special event. That said, if you have a philosophical issue with the push present, explain this to your partner—just in case all her friends give her gifts, there won't be room for any misinterpretation.

PUSH PRESENTS UNDER $100:

- Baby charm necklaces or bracelets
- Personalized sterling silver birth necklace
- Engraved picture frame with a picture of her and her pregnant belly
- Necklace, bracelet, or earrings with the baby's birthstone
- Sleep

ENAMEL ENGRAVED BABY SHOE CHARMS: These range from the low hundreds to thousand of dollars. Do an online search for "enamel baby shoes" and you'll get a good sense of what I'm talking about. If you happen to buy online, make sure to read the return policy. She might love the idea, but not the gift.

ENGRAVED GIFTS: If you're buying something expensive but are not quite sure if she'll love it, wait until she sees it, and then engrave it. When you give it to her, tell her you wanted to wait for the birth so you could engrave the date. Once you engrave it there is typically no returning it.

A way to economize is to combine the push present with some other gift-giving occasion. It gives a "big gift" much more meaning. You can make it a surprise, or plan it as a couple's project during the last trimester. Keep in mind that shopping for jewelry allows you to say and do things you can't usually say or do. She might be too happy and distracted to be pissed off with you.

When it comes to how much to spend—you can spend less than $100 or more than $1,000. Take baby bootie charms for example (charms are little pendants attached to a necklace or bracelet—think Monopoly pieces). Some charms cost under a hundred dollars; other charms may cost you in the thousands.

One of the coolest things I've seen are little silver coin-like disks that have the baby's name engraved on them. The charms attach to a necklace/bracelet, and you can add more charms as you have more kids. If you're on a tight budget, go to a bead store with her and make something together. You can also find birthstones that are extremely reasonable. If you're not sure what to get, call a maternity store and ask for advice from the manager or owner. (They might even sell something that will work.)

Guide to Birthstones

The following is a guide to birthstones, including the type and color of the stone. If you're on a budget, consider getting a stone that has the same color and features without the high price tag (for example, instead of a diamond, get cubic zirconia). You can also get something that has little bits of the stone instead of a big rock (that can cut the cost substantially).

Month	Birthstone	Color
January	Garnet	Deep Red
February	Amethyst	Purple
March	Aquamarine	Pale Blue
April	Diamond	White, Clear
May	Emerald	Green
June	Pearl	White or Purple
July	Ruby	Red
August	Peridot, Sardonyx	Pale Green
September	Sapphire	Deep Blue
October	Opal, Pink Tourmaline	Multicolor, Pink
November	Citrine, Yellow Topaz	Yellow
December	Blue Topaz, Turquoise	Blue

She doesn't actually have to push to get the present. Women who have C-section deliveries definitely qualify for the push present. I couldn't imagine still having a wife or girlfriend after telling her, "It's a push present—did you push? It's not called a C-section present, is it?"

THE BOTTOM LINE:

If she wants a push present, never tell her you want a present too (unless you're wearing a protective shield around your testicles).

Tip #55

DOING THE LITTLE THINGS: And Eating, Drinking, and Behaving as If You're Pregnant

THE TIP:

The little things will have a huge impact.

THE STORY:

I do projects around the house, but the little stuff is not my area of expertise. When she was pregnant, I would focus on the small things—like not only folding her laundry, but bringing it upstairs and putting it away too. From time to time, I'd bring home a magazine she likes. Every woman has similar "small things" that she appreciates. I found the smallest things would go a long way. It's amazing how big of a reaction I could get from doing something like putting away clothes. I don't think she knew I could do it. The only problem is that now she knows I'm capable.

—AJ, son 18 months

* * *

I titled this tip "Doing the Little Things," but it could also mean changing your ways or making sacrifices— they all accomplish the same

I decided to give up all the food she couldn't eat, the alcohol, and other recreational habits that don't go with being pregnant.

—Mike (son 3 months)

thing. All she wants is to feel appreciated and understood, and the littlest things can make a huge impression.

And really, it's not like we have to do that much while she's going through this. We satisfy some cravings, move something heavy, and go to doctor's appointments, but that's pretty much it. We don't have to sleep on our side or get hemorrhoids (at least some of us). We can eat steak tartare, drink a fifth of Jack, wear our old pants, stay out until five in the morning, hang out in smoky bars, travel at will, ride roller coasters, bungee jump, and get shaken up in those rides that simulate a high-speed adventure until you vomit. We can do everything we used to do before she got pregnant. But she can't.

She's tired, uncomfortable, sometimes nauseous, and dealing with all the emotions that come with pregnancy. Making some kind of change and doing ever so little shows her that you're trying to be supportive. But beyond that, it helps you stay connected with her throughout the pregnancy. Because we don't feel the physical parts, it's easy to forget. Doing something out of the ordinary reminds us of what's coming. Not only will something like cleaning the house help her feel supported and impress her, it will prove to be the ultimate aphrodisiac (see Tip #57).

Following are some little things you can do to help:

Don't come home drunk if your wife likes to drink. Whatever she is not allowed to do during pregnancy, she does not want to hear about you doing.

—*Jason (son 8 weeks)*

- Avoid eating things that she can't eat.
- Avoid alcohol, cigarettes, and illegal drugs.
- Avoid caffeinated beverages.
- Gain 30 pounds (just to show her you're totally committed).
- Gain 10 pounds (just to show her you're partially committed).
- Wear an empathy belly (they actually make these things).
- Don't go out without her if she's too tired (and don't make her feel bad about it).
- Ask her what movie she wants to see instead of forcing your choice.
- Clean up around the house (a little bit goes a long way).
- Do the dishes (but load the dishwasher properly—see Tip #46).
- Cook for her. For recipes, Google "Easy (fill in the blank with name of dish you want to prepare").
- Go shopping with her for clothes and baby stuff.
- Take a prenatal yoga class with her.
- Massage a body part of hers you don't usually touch.
- Read this book (or one of her books).
- Fold laundry (watch out for her underwear, it can have stuff).
- Take pictures of her belly and give them to her as a gift.
- Take an interest in her belly (listen to it, rub it, draw pictures on it).

- Get her a gift card or a small present.
- Get her flowers or a card.
- Listen to her when you don't usually listen.
- Allow her to win every argument.
- Do whatever the hell she asks you to do (at least for 40 weeks).

THE BOTTOM LINE:
She'll fall over in shock and in love when you do the little things...

8

PREGNANT SEX

Having It, Not Having It, Fantasizing about Having It

Tip #56
PREGNANT SEX 101: The 18-Inch Penis Question and More

THE TIP:
You want to get out of there right when she reaches *that* point....

THE STORY:
This is really embarrassing—but, you know how a guy has to be very adventurous when you're big and pregnant? My husband was nice enough to try and pleasure me by going down there. I didn't know that

I had poor control of my urinary tract muscles, and in the middle of the culmination, I accidentally peed in his mouth. It was a good amount of pee. He was really sweet about it—I mean *very* sweet. The whole time he was telling me that it was alright and not to worry because he knew that I was really so embarrassed. He just rinsed out his mouth and brushed his teeth and made sure I was okay. This tip is good advice for everyone.

—Gloria, daughter 2 years

* * *

The big question: *Will having sex hurt the baby?*

We know in theory that the penis can't reach the baby, but it's hard to believe in the moment. So to address this question, I asked a leading doctor with over thirty years of experience in the field the following question: *If someone reading this has an 18-inch penis, would having sex hurt the baby?*

The doctor's response was, "First of all, this reader must have an enormous imagination to go along with his penis. But the rule is: If it's uncomfortable, don't do it." He wouldn't suggest using large sex toys, but a large penis shouldn't pose a problem. Just make sure she's not uncomfortable. He went on to explain that if someone is concerned, bring it up with your caregiver. These questions are normal, and doctors and other care providers are comfortable addressing them.

Assuming sex is medically safe, the idea that your penis is a few inches from your baby's head can be a bit deflating, distracting, and a total turnoff. So, get the thought of your penis being near the baby's head out of your head. I know it's hard to *not* think of your penis being close to the baby because you keep reading "penis near baby," but let it go. I only say it because *you are not* going to hurt the baby.

When having sex, do not think about the BV (birthing vagina). Focus solely on the SV (sex vagina). In fact, nature designed the SV to keep a couple sexually connected during pregnancy. The SV is built for pregnant sex. As big as you might be, the baby is well protected from the outside world (your penis included). The mucous plug, the uterus (the strongest organ in the female body), and the amniotic sac are there to protect the baby. As for the fear of being grabbed by the baby, the baby is in his secure bubble. Some guys get freaked out about finishing inside; but again, it's not getting near the baby. The biggest risk of injury as a result of pregnant sex? It's her falling off, knocking the wind out of you, or smacking you when you playfully grab her nipples (see Tip #57).

Of course, any sex questions need to be addressed to your caregiver. Go to a doctor's appointment and ask when your partner is out of the room (if she or you are uncomfortable asking together). You can also call your caregiver's office and talk to any of the doctors on call. Unless your doctor says, "NO SEX FOR YOU" (like the Soup Nazi in *Seinfeld*), there should

ORAL SEX WARNING:
Never blow air inside her vagina—this can cause an embolism and the baby and mother could die. If you happen to be the guy whose signature move is blowing air inside her vagina, please pick another place to blow.

be sex for you (assuming she's willing, interested, and able to have it).

What medical issues might shut down your sex life? A medical condition like placenta previa (when the placenta is located on or near the cervix) or something like preterm labor, a history of miscarriages, bleeding, leaking, or a cervical condition can shut down the sex factory. If she has a normal-risk pregnancy and experiences something out of the norm like bleeding, leaking, cramping, or contracting, ask the doctor if sex can be had. And if the vagina is off-limits, there are other things you can do besides penetration.

Assuming you have clearance to enter the sex arena, appreciate that things will change. She might not be able to do what she used to do. She might fall off, roll around, feel uncomfortable, get more turned on, get less turned on, have more lubrication or less, or her body could react in ways that surprise her. She might be a different woman in the bedroom. You won't know until you get there. How to get there is addressed in Tip #57.

THE BOTTOM LINE:

The pregnant vagina can be fiercely intimidating and unpredictable at times, but we need to persevere—we *must* persevere, we *can* persevere.

Tip #57
A GUIDE TO PREGNANT SEX (VERSION 1.0): The Essentials Every Man Needs to Know

THE TIP:

1. Make her feel like you're nuts about her.
2. Always be helpful and caring.
3. Make up stuff as you go.

THE STORY:

1. I've learned that if a woman knows that you're attracted to her she will get extremely turned on by this—even a pregnant woman. I've also learned that all women are self-conscious, especially when big and pregnant. You have to make them feel like you are crazy nuts about them all the time. Don't be timid when having sex. Do it how you used to do it. Don't change your style or she'll interpret it as you not being as attracted or turned on. Go at it.

2. Seducing her isn't always about touching her in certain places. For example, when my wife was shellacking cabinets with a regular varnish—the kind of varnish that can give your kids three heads—I found an organic varnish that wouldn't harm the fetus. She thought it was the sweetest, most caring thing in the world. I mean, she was so happy that we had mind-blowing pregnant sex. Helping her out and showing you care is a huge turn-on.

3. The final suggestion is to make up stuff that will make her feel incredibly attractive and sexy. One time I created an intimate moment with candles and music and told my wife that I have a secret fetish for pregnant women. I told her that I fantasize about pregnant women and visit pregnancy porn sites on the Internet. I asked her if she could indulge me just this one time. It worked one time. The next day, she realized I was full of it, but she forgave me.

—Danny, father of four

✳ ✳ ✳

As part of my research for the book, I interviewed more than one hundred pregnant men and women from around the world and asked them to open their bedroom doors and share the truth about having (or not having) pregnant sex. Below are some of the best answers from my first round of questioning. I say that this is only the first round because I'd like your help with the Dad's Pregnant Too Pregnant Sex Project. If you have stories, tips, or suggestions, please forward them to me via www.DadsPregnant.com.

Before sharing the pregnant sex data, I want to touch on the frequency-of-sex results. In general, most couples' rate of pregnant sex decreased as the pregnancy progressed. There are too many variables that affect the results to include them (nausea, sensitivity, medical issues, guys getting freaked out, etc). I can sum it up like this: If you're having sex right now, you'll most likely continue having sex throughout the pregnancy. (And if you're having sex right now, it's amazing that you can keep this book steady and continue to read.) If you're not having much sex right now, then you'll continue to not have much sex. And if you've had a lot of sex before and aren't having it now, there might be some things you can do to increase your chances (see below), assuming you're not the one rejecting your pregnant partner. And now the results…

BEST POSITION FOR PREGNANT SEX?
- Spooning.
- Woman on the side.
- Doggie style (Some women listed it as worst, too).
- Woman on top.
- Keeping it simple.
- A pillow under the belly right by the pelvic bone (Be careful when she starts to show or when the

baby starts to move, as her pelvic area gets a bit tender).

- Woman laying in bed as usual but man underneath hips; he does all the moving (also good for post C-section).

WORST POSITION FOR PREGNANT SEX?

- Missionary—it doesn't work.
- Anything requiring balance.
- Anything too bouncy.
- Anything involving too much flexibility.
- Doggie style can be uncomfortable at times.
- Woman acting as dominatrix on top (Hard to carry off the stern thing when wobbling and rolling off…).
- All positions (some women are tender down there now and sex can become a turn off).

WHAT CAN A MAN DO TO INCREASE HIS CHANCES OF HAVING SEX?

- Don't get her pregnant (most popular answer).
- Make her feel like a goddess and be experimental.
- Massage and rub her shoulders, feet…you name it.
- Run a bubble bath for her (not too hot).
- Tell her she still looks amazing, hot, and sexy.
- Make her feel important and absolutely gorgeous.
- Always think of her needs first. All else will follow.
- Do all the chores so that she has energy for sex.
- Be patient and sensual.
- Make an effort to kiss her neck and softly touch her.

- Put on some nice music, and go with the flow.
- Try kissing her and saying, "Let's have sex, hot lady."
- Help out with child #1 so she's not tired and pissed off.
- Be very nice to her.
- Get her ice cream when she wants it.
- Don't ask for it (or beg for it or demand it).
- Nothing. If she doesn't want it, you'll only aggravate her by asking.
- Do not push it. (Men have no idea what it's like to be pregnant. Women already have enough demands to have you make demands.)
- Make sure she knows that she is the only one for you and that she's still attractive.
- Try sex in the morning—she's a lot less likely to be too tired.
- Masturbate…it makes you less desperate.

TIPS OR SUGGESTIONS FOR SATISFYING A PREGNANT WOMAN IN BED?

- Take more time for foreplay.
- Massage her before having sex.
- Brush your teeth. Bad breath can be a huge deal breaker when she's extra-sensitive to smells.
- Have oral sex.
- Be very gentle and avoid touching the breasts at all in the first trimester (excruciating pain doesn't usually put her in the mood).

- Let her do what she wants to do in bed (no forcing her).
- Engage in standard cuddling.
- Find out what her favorite part of her body is. (It can change when she is pregnant.) Make sure you always start by making her feel wanted and beautiful.
- Ask her what she wants you to do—her desires have probably changed and she may have very specific instructions.
- Don't be freaked out by the baby and her changing shape.
- Treat sex like a fun experimental thing rather than an inconvenience.
- Give her whatever she wants.
- Be willing to do lots of work, especially toward the end!
- Make her feel beautiful all the time.

WHAT SHOULD A MAN *NEVER* DO WITH HIS PREGNANT WIFE/PARTNER IN BED?

- Blow in her vagina—this can cause an embolism and the baby and mother can die!
- Talk about her size.
- Grab her nipples (or bite too hard).
- Tell her she's fat.
- Squeeze pressure points in her ankle which may send her into labor.
- Tell her she's too big for sex.
- Make her feel bad if there's a little blood or odor.

- Ask her if she wants anal sex or wants to give you oral sex.
- Bug her for sex or make her feel guilty for not having it.
- Watch sporting events and put moves on simultaneously.
- Assume she wants it.
- Use the words *fat* and *hormonal*.
- Say that the baby moving around is interfering too much to have sex.
- Try new things without asking first. (It's a lot easier to get hurt with a full uterus!)
- Expect her to just do anything at any time.
- Have rough sex with her (without asking first).
- Do anything she isn't up for.
- Become impatient with her.
- Put her into any position that makes her feel uncomfortable.
- Rub her belly and say "Wow" like you can't believe she's *that* enormous.
- Get upset if something leaks or squirts.

MOST HILARIOUS OR AWKWARD SEX MOMENT?
- "I farted."
- "It was a month and a half before our due date and while we were fooling around he stopped me and asked why I was drooling all over his chest— I wasn't, I was lactating!"

- "I would want it more than he did. He couldn't keep up with me."
- "The baby kicked while in missionary. My fiancé could feel her kick him too."
- "I had an overall lack of coordination as the pregnancy progressed—we had klutzy lovemaking."
- "When I was pregnant with my second, I was huge and knocked the wind out of him with my belly."
- "The baby started moving during the deed—we kept going though."
- "I was sick at the sight and smell of his semen."
- "I got leg cramps in the middle of it."
- "The baby would use my cervix as a trampoline and he would enter at the same time."
- "As I was trying to get comfy near the end, I rolled off a few times."
- "I wasn't able to move when I was about 38 weeks pregnant. I was huge and there was not too much I could do from my end."
- "I would wake up extremely horny. I practically jumped on him. This is a big deal as I have *never* been a morning sex person."
- "I peed in his mouth."

THE BOTTOM LINE:

Please send me your pregnant sex tips, stories, and suggestions so I can include them in the next edition. Send them via www.DadsPregnant.com

Tip #58

MEN WHO DON'T WANT SEX: If You're Rejecting Your Pregnant Partner

THE TIP:

If you don't want sex with her while she's pregnant, make sure to help her feel beautiful and desirable.

THE STORY:

We had a lot of sex at the beginning of the pregnancy. As the months progressed, the sex slowed down. During the last couple of months, he no longer wanted it at all. I know it was awkward for him (I once got a leg cramp in the middle of it) and that he was concerned for the baby, but his lack of interest made me feel ugly and bad about myself. Even if he didn't want to have sex, it would have been nice if he found other ways to make me feel attractive and loved. It didn't have to be a sexual thing; he could have planned something like a romantic dinner for no reason just to show me he still cared.

—Lesha, sons 8 months and 2½ years

＊ ＊ ＊

We used to have sex every day before I got pregnant. Since I got pregnant, it's been gradually less and less. I'm starting to feel resentful toward him because I have needs too. It took two to make this baby, and he still wants me to pleasure him.

—Claire (37 weeks pregnant)

After years of always wanting to have sex and not always getting it (at least that's how it worked for me), some guys don't want to have sex with a pregnant woman. They just can't do it. It's just one of the phenomena of being an expectant father. It might be a fear of hurting the baby. It might be your partner's physical appearance. (Women don't want to hear this, but it can happen.) The huge changes, long hours working to get ready for the arrival, or mounting anxiety might shut down your sex drive. If you don't want it and your partner does, be sensitive to how this is interpreted in her world.

Pregnant woman are not especially good with rejection. In general, no one loves rejection. And a woman who is uncomfortable in her Expectant Mother Thong (see Tip #42: The Hormonal Pregnant Woman) is especially vulnerable. She sees rejection as something being wrong with her. She sees you as not being attracted to her. She sees you as being detached and uninterested. It's more than the sex.

So, if you're not in the mood, it's crucial for you to explain the circumstances behind the sexual rejection. If it's too sensitive to share with her or if you're not sure why you feel this way, just tell her it makes you uncomfortable, but it has nothing to do with her not being beautiful. Blame it on being weirded out by having a baby so close to your penis. Whatever you do, just make a big effort to stay physically connected and show her that you still love her. Hug her more, kiss her more, rub her down more, get her flowers or a gift—do something so that she will never doubt how much you love her and care about her.

NO SEX WARNING

If you find that you're not as physically attracted to your pregnant partner, recognize that this may have nothing to do with her body. Yes, there are physical changes, but on some level, her new look is a constant reminder of a lifetime of responsibility and huge changes coming your way. (By the way, they're great changes.) That's one reason some guys freak out and distance themselves (emotionally or physically).

A pregnant woman is beautiful. She's a different kind of woman than whom you married. It's a temporary change, but it's a change you can't fight. Give yourself time to adjust to the idea of her being different. And if you still can't see it, instead of shutting down, figure out why you're feeling this way. If it's too sensitive to discuss with her, consider enlisting

Attention Rejected Expectant Fathers: If your partner is the one who doesn't want sex with you, revisit Tip #16: The Rejected Expectant Father. Also consider discussing the suggestions in Tip #57 with her. This might help you figure out how to seduce her and get her in the mood.

the help of a professional. Once you can reframe these issues, her new look should only make her that much more attractive to you.

And if you don't want to have sex, and she wants some action, get creative and find other ways to please her. I guarantee that at some point during the pregnancy (or your life), she's done it for you.

THE BOTTOM LINE:
If you lose your sex drive, don't let it drive you away. Get creative and find new ways to make her feel beautiful and desirable.

Tip #59
MEN WHO HAVE SEX ALONE: How Pregnant Women Feel about Porn

THE TIP:
Some pregnant women don't like it when men look at attractive naked or half-naked women who aren't pregnant. Don't argue.

THE STORY:
A neighbor gave me some magazines and left an *FHM* magazine for my husband, which I put straight into the garbage bin. (I used to look like the girls in those magazines but I obviously looked nothing like that anymore!) Anyway, I told him that the neighbor gave

me some magazines, but I threw the *FHM* away. He then went on to ask me why I tossed it and argued with me because he never goes out of his way to buy these kinds of magazines for himself and would have liked to flip through it! I stormed off in a huff because I honestly felt threatened and jealous. Here I am carrying his baby and he doesn't want to make love to me at all, but it's okay for him to look at girls in expensive underwear that I could never wear because I'm having his baby!

—Claire, 37 weeks pregnant

* * *

I'll just jump headfirst into this one—some of you reading this have a special appreciation for porn. For those of you who don't love porn, you might enjoy soft porn (publications thinly veiled as men's magazines).

While you might love it, some women have a huge problem with this. A lot of it comes from the fact that many pregnant women are uncomfortable in their thongs (see Tip #42: The Hormonal Pregnant Woman). The idea of you looking at another woman and getting turned on can be threatening (especially if you're not having sex with your pregnant partner). Whether it's a men's magazine or a hardcore website, when it comes

My wife knows that I have the propensity to look at porn online—she gives me that. She just looks at me and rolls her eyes. We used to watch it together so she understands.

—Loving Porn-Consuming Husband

to focusing your sexual energy elsewhere, it's impossible to explain to the love of your life that what you're doing is a harmless outlet that has nothing to do with her and your sex life (or lack thereof). By definition, if she's harmed, it's not harmless.

I'm not promoting or condemning porn—I'm just saying if you use porn, don't be so careless that you get "caught in the act" or leave traces on your computer, iPod, cell phone, or in your bedroom (and if you're concealing that much porn you might have an addiction). Women (pregnant or not) discovering porn and freaking out after finding it is one of the most frequently written-about issues in my syndicated advice column (HelpMeHarlan.com). Yes, loving, caring, monogamous men do look at porn, but you don't want to have to explain this to a blindsided pregnant woman. The advice is simple:

1. Do not let it happen.

2. If caught, don't fight it.

If she finds out that you're using porn, expect her to be upset, to doubt your level of attraction to her, and to feel betrayed. Don't fight it. She might think you're cheating. She might yell, cry, or just leave you (yes, it happens). Most women (pregnant or not) don't see how porn and masturbation can be an outlet for stress and anxiety—they see it as a threat or reflective of your lack of satisfaction or commitment. What women may not realize is that some guys have been consuming porn and masturbating long before marriage. This doesn't make it okay, but the point is that it's habitual and can have little to do with his level of commitment or desire for his partner. Sure, there are healthier ways to relieve stress, but women aren't as threatened by a guy participating in a fantasy bowling league as opposed to a guy watching fantasy bowling porn. (I might find that a little strange too.)

Should you have to explain the unexplainable, tell your partner that this is more about stress and anxiety than the images on the screen. If she can't get over it, get counseling together. Make sure she knows you love her, and don't give her more reasons to doubt your commitment. If you want to stop using but can't, or if she wants to you to stop but you can't, seek support and treatment. While you might think porn is harmless, the moment it causes harm it stops being harmless.

THE BOTTOM LINE:

While there are millions of men in happy, healthy, and loving relationships who consume pornography, no pregnant partner who isn't into porn or isn't aware of her partner's use should have to discover this while pregnant.

9

SHOPPING FOR BABY

Something So Little Needs So Much

Tip #60
SHOPPING FOR BABY: How Could Something So Little Need So Much?

THE TIP:

Go to the store and register so when people want to get something for you they'll know what to buy.

THE STORY:

A lot of people are willing to help out, but they don't know what to get us. We're having a shower soon so we are in the process of registering. It's overwhelming how much stuff there is online. I find it helps to see it and touch it. This weekend, I spent over four hours shopping—two at Wal-Mart and two and a half at Babies 'R' Us. We were pre-registering—and no, this isn't registering; it's what happens *before* you register. I have never felt more lost and overwhelmed in four aisles of a store. Do we need this? Which bottles are the right bottles? She looks at me like, "I don't know which ones to get." And I'm thinking the same thing. Another suggestion is to pack a snack and water— you don't want to have a hungry pregnant wife on your hands.

—*Scott, 6 months pregnant*

* * *

Welcome to the baby superstore. Please let me show you around. Here you will find the: *strollers, car seats, infant seats, cribs, bassinettes, co-sleepers, monitors, baby carriers, diapers, diaper bags, diaper dispensers, diaper rash creams, baby wipes, changing pads, changing tables, baby furniture sets, rockers, pacifiers, bottles, nipples, blankets, swaddlers, lotions, rectal thermometers, swings, bedding sets, layettes (the baby's first clothing, bedding, and essentials for the first three months), hats, socks, shoes, towels, wash-cloths, baby bathtubs, baby soaps, bathtub toys,*

Going to Babies 'R' Us for a woman is *rubbing alcohols, cotton balls* like going to Best Buy for a man. *(to clean the belly button),*
—Cathy (sons 4 months and 3½ years) *anti-gas medications, nasal*

aspirators, infant medicines, infant nail clippers, hairbrushes, combs, tweezers, brushes to clean bottles, toys, stuffed animals, rattles, bouncy seats, kids' CDs, (if nursing) breast milk storage bottles, breast pumps, and much, much more!

It's easy to see that it can all be so overwhelming. So here are some tips to keep in mind while buying things for baby:

- First locate the gliders/rocking chairs. They are a great place to sit while she shops.
- Find something that interests you so you don't go out of your mind (focus on the stroller, baby gates, or a construction project that can engage you).
- Bring food in case she gets hungry (but don't eat it all first).
- Shop at the houses of friends and family. We borrowed a stroller, the co-sleeper, the baby carrier, baby clothing, maternity clothes, and stuff they didn't even know we took (we moved *very* fast).
- Don't open the box until you need it (this way you can still return it).
- *Save all receipts* (you'll need them if you break something during assembly).
- Know the return policy. Some stores have limited windows because babies outgrow stuff so fast.
- Get storage containers (great for holding all the little things).
- Let an expert assemble the crib unless you're a

My wife hates to shop. We only order things online.

—*Todd (son 4 months)*

REQUIRED READING:
Baby Bargains by Denise and Alan Fields: www.babybargains.com. This *amazing* book will answer most of your questions. Sign up for their newsletter and get alerts on recalls or products mentioned in the book. The book hits on all the major purchases and offers pros, cons, and inside information on the most essential products.

handyman (build this into the cost when budgeting).

- Always ask if there's a coupon when checking out. (Sometimes a sales-clerk will pull one out of thin air.)
- If people buy gifts you won't use for several months, consider returning them for store credit. Buy an item when you need it.
- Kids outgrow expensive clothes as fast as inexpensive clothes (sucks, I know).
- Shopping with grandparents can be cost-effective.
- Don't buy the big-ticket items right away (coworkers might pool their money and buy you a ridiculous stroller).
- Buy the essentials and wait to get everything else as you need it.
- Take advantage of free shipping and bulk discounts when ordering online.

- Avoid paying sales tax by buying some things online and having the heavy stuff shipped to your door (diapers, formula, big-ticket items).
- A burping up, spitting up, peeing, and pooping baby will have just as much fun sleeping on and staining the inexpensive bedding.
- If you're putting together a crib, car seat, or anything that swings, moves, makes noise, or needs batteries, *read the directions first* (this one is hard).
- Over time, all diaper dispenser systems will smell like a Porta-Potty on a hot summer's day.
- Register everything you buy with the manufacturer so that you will receive recall messages or other essential information.

PREGNANCY Q & A:

QUESTION: The biggest argument or point of contention while shopping?
ANSWER: He wanted to read the *Consumer Reports* reviews about *every* item we registered for and I just wanted to go with the things my friends had recommended. (Jenn, daughter 22 months)
My husband always looked at the cheapest thing and thought it would be fine. It didn't matter if it was highly recommended or not. He wasn't thinking safety first. (Megan, daughter 11 months)

- If getting things secondhand, make sure they're safe. (Never buy a used car seat or a crib that has a history that can't be verified.) Check the recall list by visiting: www.recalls.gov.

THE BOTTOM LINE:
It's mind boggling how someone under 10 pounds can need so much, but it will never make you happier than to watch your son or daughter use it all (well, maybe not the diaper dispenser).

Tip #61
THE EMOTIONAL PURCHASE: You'll Cry When You See the Bill

THE TIP:
As a rule, avoid making emotional purchases (with a few exceptions).

THE STORY:
My wife has always been an emotional shopper. There were several times when she wanted to make an emotional purchase for the baby. One incident that sticks out was a $2,000 bassinette—something that would last only a couple months. Even the less expensive bassinette was $500. We avoided that purchase altogether. It's not tough for me to say "No." I figure if I'm having a baby girl I need to get used to saying it!

If you think your wife can spend, your wife and daughter combined can spend enough to bankrupt you. If there is practical use for something, a "No" can turn into a "Yes." It's the difference between what we *want* and what we *need*. From time to time, we do indulge in the wants. When she was pregnant she wanted a piece of jewelry that represented the circle of life, so after our daughter was born, she "bought" it and presented the jewelry to her mom. Buying the stroller was an exercise in wearing me down. It was like the movie *Groundhog Day*—over and over and over again until we finally got the one I swore we would never get. My wife jokes that I'm the meanest man on the planet. My motto: Take care of the pennies and the pounds take care of themselves.

—Kevin, daughter 3 months

✳ ✳ ✳

If you have an endless budget, this tip doesn't apply to you (read Tip #62: The Perfect Stroller). If you are on a budget, shopping for the baby can be an emotional experience. Seeing the credit card statement is the moment when most men break down in tears. There's a lot to buy and emotions are tied to them all (even a rectal thermometer). From the bedding to the crib to the

Watch her like a hawk; salespeople know how easy it is to sell expensive bedding to a pregnant lady. They can convince you to buy a lot of things that you don't know whether you'll need yet.

—Emily (mother of two)

stroller to the car seat—if you're not careful you can easily spend a small fortune.

Often it's the man who ends up playing the role of the bad guy. Here's the problem: She's physically and emotionally transformed and busy spending all her time researching a purchase. When she's ready to pull the trigger, in walks the guy complaining that it costs too much or reporting that *Consumer Reports* says it's the wrong choice. Then it can become a fight. And when it comes to fighting with a pregnant woman, even if you win, you feel terrible.

Here are some things that can prevent her from getting sad and you feeling bad:

- Figure out what you need versus what you want. Create a NEEDS column and a WANTS column. Stick to what you need and wait to see if you can get what you want as a gift. The emotional purchase can wait.

- Set a budget early, figure out what you can afford, and then find a way to stick to it. If you have a budget in place, you can refer to it when her emotions (or yours) run high. Blame it on the budget.

- Be involved early on in the process. This means having a sense of what things cost and why they cost that much. For example, not all strollers are created equal. The more expensive strollers might last longer than the less expensive ones. The price doesn't tell the entire story.

- When it comes to *great* deals, make sure the company can deliver and that what they're delivering is safe. Since we had our first baby, I've watched one baby furniture store chain go out of business and another change owners. One company would take orders and *never* deliver the cribs. Investigate their customer service policies before making the purchase (do an online search and post comments in new parent community forums).

THE BOTTOM LINE:
The emotional purchase cryfecta (like a trifecta):
1. The salesperson cries because her commission is so huge.
2. Your pregnant partner cries because the nursery is so beautiful.
3. You cry because you had to sell a limb to pay for it all.

Tip #62
THE PERFECT STROLLER(S): They Can't Go 55 Miles per Hour, But They Should, Given Some of the Prices

THE TIP:
All strollers break down differently. Once you figure out how to make one collapse, help out your fellow man.

THE STORY:

Shopping for the stroller was one of the most memorable experiences. You walk down the aisle and see a row of guys struggling with the strollers trying to collapse them, but no two collapse the same way. You see some guys just standing there staring blankly at the stroller. Meanwhile other guys are kicking, struggling, pushing, and pulling until the strollers break down or just break. There are so many different levers and buttons. Once I figured out how to collapse a stroller, I would walk down the aisle and help out other guys struggling with them. How a stroller collapses was a factor in what we decided to buy. We ended up with two strollers. We went with the smallest stroller that fit in my trunk and a jogging stroller for home. Honestly, we still can't figure out how to break down the jogging stroller.

—Chris, son 22 months

＊＊＊

The 1800s marked the industrial revolution. The early 2000s will be known throughout history as the stroller revolution. We've come a long way from the umbrella stroller that was standard issue when we were strolling with our parents.

Things to keep in mind: Make sure he can use it. Can he figure out how to open it and close it? Is he too tall to reach the handles? Make sure it can take a beating. Strollers get bashed around a lot.

—Emily (mother of two)

Top engineering, research and development, and state of the art materials have thrust us into the future. Some (who, I don't know) would call it the golden age of strollers.

Strollers vary in function, style, and price. You can get a stroller for $10 or one for over $1,000. The perfect stroller is like the perfect pair of jeans—it's a personal choice based on a list of very specific criteria. There are some real differences between the most inexpensive strollers and the most expensive ones. Adjustable versus nonadjustable handles, plastic versus rubber wheels, storage capacity, and versatility are some things to consider.

When you walk into the stroller showroom, it's important to arrive with a budget, specific needs, and suggestions of like-minded friends. Bring the *Baby Bargains* book or a *Consumer Reports* with you. Be in control. Without a budget and guidelines in mind, it's like walking into a car dealership that sells Mercedes and Ford Escorts on the same lot. The emotions can push you into buying a stroller that's beyond your needs or means. Some things to keep in mind when shopping:

- Know your budget. (Again, discuss this with each other before setting foot in the store.)
- Is the stroller safe and durable? (Check out the *Baby Bargains* book.)
- How does it feel during test driving? (Put something in it that weighs similar to a baby to get the feel for turning, braking, and acceleration.)

- Do you kick the wheels while strolling? (Some guys are taller than their partners.)
- Do you have to bend over to push it? (That will kill you.)
- Does it hurt your back, shoulders, or extremities to push? (Adjustable arms can be helpful.)
- How much space is in the cargo area beneath the basket? (If there isn't room to hold the bag, you'll be holding the bag.)
- Are you going to be off-roading or mostly mall strolling? (Sidewalks cause wear and tear.)
- Is it easy to clean and machine washable? (Spilled milk can stink. I have to wash ours once every couple of months.)
- Is the size right? (Some strollers are too wide for store aisles, not unlike Hummers on the road.)
- What matters most to you (or her)—vanity or functionality?

The last thing you probably want to hear about buying a stroller is that it's a good idea to get two strollers. That's what we did. One is lightweight (and was a gift) that we use for travel and keep in the trunk. The other is bigger and a little more expensive (great for city strolling). Our only regret is that the seat on our big stroller doesn't turn around. We can't see our daughter's face while strolling. I think looking at her would have cost us another $400. So, instead, we carry a picture of her and look at it while we stroll.

THE STROLLER EXPERT

To help address the stroller question, I tapped into the mind of a stroller expert I came across while running an errand for my wife. (I had to buy some bottles.) I overheard this guy talking to a woman about strollers and was blown away by how much he knew. He could have been publisher of *Stroller Monthly* magazine (if there was such a magazine). After the woman finished speaking with him, I asked him if he could address some questions for the book. Here's the dialogue that ensued:

QUESTION: *What is the biggest mistake men make when shopping for strollers?*

ANSWER: Expectant fathers often downplay how often they will be using the stroller and defer to their wives, thinking that the stroller should better suit her. But, a 6'4" father and a 4'11" mother cannot comfortably use the same stroller unless the handlebar adjusts for user height.

QUESTION: *Your tips for shopping for a stroller on a budget?*

ANSWER: Always consider your current needs and how they might change with the addition of a child. Ask yourself where you will be using the stroller most often, as terrain determines wheel type, which will affect the weight of the stroller. If you jog, ask yourself if you will continue to jog after the baby is born and if you will be in the market for a jogging stroller. Also take into account your body type versus your wife's body type and the height factor. If you are on a budget, buy one or two quality aluminum-framed strollers (one for rough terrain or jogging and one to travel with) instead of buying a cheap plastic stroller, which will likely need to be replaced after very little real use.

QUESTION: *Tips for shopping with a limitless budget?*
ANSWER: If you have a limitless budget, treat yourself to something top of the line and make your partner happy. That said, limit yourself to two or three good strollers per child unless you also have limitless storage space. (*Author note:* Not sure if I agree with this one.)

QUESTION: *Ever seen a couple get in a fight while shopping?*
ANSWER: Yes, although I can't recall any specific details. Often, if the husband appears to be apathetic or bummed because he's missing the game, his wife will pick up on it. On the flip side, his wife should be concerned with more than just the color or brand name of the stroller and take into account her husband's concerns about mechanics and warranty.

QUESTION: *Any essentials guys shopping with their pregnant partners should keep in mind?*

ANSWER: Guys need to remain logical and focused, as their pregnant partners are often emotional time bombs.

THE BOTTOM LINE:
Safety, comfort (yours, hers, and baby's), warranty, and price do matter. If opting for a less stylish stroller, consider aftermarket rims, a subwoofer, and a rear spoiler.

Tip #63
THE CRIB, FURNITURE, AND NURSERY: No Assembly Required…If You Pay Them to Assemble It

THE TIP:
Test it before you allow your wife and baby to use it.

THE STORY:
I've always wanted an old fashioned rocking chair— not one of those padded gliders, but a real rocking chair. As a gift, my husband surprised me by getting the rocking chair I had always wanted. It was one of those chairs that he was supposed to construct. He put it together and had it all ready for me. The first night home, when the baby got up in the middle of the night, I picked her up and walked over to the chair to feed her. The rocking chair was gorgeous. I went to sit in the chair and all of sudden I fell flat on the floor. I fell

down hard and fast and screamed as loud as I could scream. I broke my fall with my shoulder so I wouldn't drop my daughter. There was wood everywhere—I'm not kidding, it was straight out of a cartoon. That was the last thing he ever built. I would never trust a changing table he constructed.

—Rebekah, daughters 2 years and 4 years

✳ ✳ ✳

The baby's room will need a crib, furniture, a rocker (or glider), a changing table, and a 42-inch flat screen TV. (Just kidding…it will need a 52-inch flat screen TV.) The big issues when it comes to these essentials are the timing, the cost, and the safety.

There are two timing issues. The first is that it sometimes takes several months from the date you order furniture until it's delivered. So, when she starts shopping during week 13, she's not just overexcited, she's making sure you get everything in time. The second issue is that when a pregnant woman's nesting instinct kicks in, she's going to want it done when she wants it done—unless you've preempted her timeline (see Tip #48)—and she will be relentless. Create a timeline for when you'll get things done before she brings it up.

When it comes to the cost, you can spend hundreds or thousands. You can get new furniture, used furniture, preassembled furniture, or furniture you need to assemble. If you're thinking of buying used furniture, make sure it's safe (check for recalls—see the sidebar). If you purchase furniture that needs to be assembled, my best advice is to pay a professional to do it (the delivery person should be trained). If it costs you $50 to make sure it's done correctly, it's a small price to pay for safety. There's no room for errors (or extra pieces) when it comes to your baby's safety. If you assemble the crib, take pictures of what the finished product is supposed to look like. Check out the furniture on the showroom floor. Take digital photos from all angles (underneath too). Even if there's a picture on the box, it's worth making sure you have some kind of visual guide to go along with the 1,421 assembly steps. If you find that you have extra pieces, don't just toss them aside. Call a professional.

When budgeting for the nursery, there are ways to spend less and still create a cool space—things like adding a wallpaper border, stenciling names with

THE TOP FIVE HIDDEN HOME HAZARDS:

(Source: U.S. Consumer Product Safety Commission, 2007)

#1 Magnets—Since 2005, there have been 1 death, 86 injuries, and 8 million toys recalled due to magnets.

#2 Recalled products—Each year there are about 400 recalls. Get dangerous products out of the home. Join the U.S. Consumer Product Safety Commission's (CPSC) "Drive to One Million" campaign and sign up for free email notifications at

THE TOP FIVE HIDDEN HOME HAZARDS: (Contd.)

https://www.cpsc.gov/cps clist.aspx. An email from CPSC is not spam—it could save a life.

#3 Tip-overs (e.g., furniture, shelves, chairs, etc.)—Average of 22 deaths per year; in 2006, 31 deaths and an estimated 3,000 injuries. Anchor your furniture to the wall or consult an expert.

#4 Windows and coverings—Average of 12 deaths annually from window cords; average

paint, printing out photos of animals and framing them, photographing the baby's body parts, or using a quilt that comes with the bedding as a wall hanging. (Quilts shouldn't be in the crib with the newborn anyway.) Before buying something, see if it can be made. If you're decorating a room before you know the baby's gender, you can use neutral colors and add gender-specific wallpaper borders, stencils, wall hangings, etc. after the baby arrives.

Regarding safety, contact a baby-proofing service and have an expert walk through your place and point out problem areas. While it's too soon to do it all, there are some things you can do now. Make sure you have a carbon monoxide detector and fire alarm inside the baby's room. If the bedroom is on a high floor, consider an escape ladder. If there are window coverings, make sure there are no strangulation hazards. Before the baby starts crawling, make sure you cover up or remove doorstops (the rubber pieces on the end can be choking hazards), cover exposed outlets, baby-proof sliding drawers, install baby gates, lower the temperature on the hot water tank, and anchor anything to the wall that can tip over and fall. When it comes to crib safety, take note of the following suggestions from the U.S. Consumer Product Safety Commission:

For cribs there should be:

- A firm, tight-fitting mattress so a baby cannot get trapped between the mattress and the crib.
- No missing, loose, broken, or improperly installed screws, brackets, or other hardware on the crib or mattress support.

THE TOP FIVE HIDDEN HOME HAZARDS: (Contd.)

of 9 deaths and an estimated 3,700 injuries to children annually from window falls.

#5 Pool and spa drains (the suction can pull small children down)— 15 injuries, 2 fatalities between 2002–2004.

- No more than 2 $^3/_8$ inches (about the width of a soda can) between crib slats so a baby's body cannot fit through the slats; no missing or cracked slats.
- No corner posts over $^1/_{16}$ inch high, so a baby's clothing cannot catch.
- No cutouts in the headboard or footboard so a baby's head cannot get trapped.

For mesh-sided cribs or playpens, look for:
- Mesh less than $^1/_4$ inch in size, smaller than the tiny buttons on a baby's clothing.
- Mesh with no tears, holes, or loose threads that could entangle a baby.
- Mesh securely attached to top rail and floor plate.
- Top rail cover with no tears or holes.
- If staples are used, they are not missing, loose, or exposed.

THE BOTTOM LINE:

When assembling things, leftover pieces are a sign that you're not good at it. (Hire a pro and sleep easy knowing everything is safe.)

Tip #64
THE CAR SEAT(S): You'll Probably Need Two (I Know, It's Ridiculous)

THE TIP:
This might be the first time you read installation directions from cover to cover. It might also be the first time you'll realize your backseat has a LATCH system.

THE STORY:
From the moment I found out we were expecting to the moment I took the infant car seat out of the box, I was adjusting to the idea of parenthood. Installing the car seat was the first time I felt like I was being a dad. I had a distinct feeling of fatherly responsibility—that I was helping this little person to be safe. After removing the seat from the box, I studied it and read the manual from cover to cover. I must have read every single word, although I did skip the German and French parts. There are a couple of different ways to install the car seat. There's the seatbelt installation and then there's the LATCH installation. I was relieved to find out that we had the LATCH system (didn't even know it when I got the car, just got lucky). I highly recommend the LATCH system. Once the seat was firmly in place, I practiced with a teddy bear that I estimated to be the same size as a baby to get a feel for the straps and buckles. I'll never forget the

image of this little teddy bear strapped in the seat with a five-point harness ready to go for a ride.

—*Josh, son 13 months*

✳ ✳ ✳

You may have been surprised to read in Tip #62 that your pregnant partner might want to buy two strollers (one for home and one for the car/travel). Well, I hate to be the one to tell you this, but she's also going to tell you that you'll need two car seats within the first year (most likely). You're probably thinking that one is enough (that's what I thought). But here's why you'll need two…

The infant seat will work for up to twelve months (up to 30 pounds and 26 inches in length). The convertible car seat (it "converts" from backward facing to forward facing) is for the next several years (up to 40 pounds). You'll want the infant seat so you can move the baby in and out of the car without waking him up (the entire infant seat snaps into the base, which stays in the car). You'll want the convertible seat once the baby outgrows the infant seat (this stays in the car). So this is why you'll actually *need* two seats (not just want them).

When it comes to installing the infant car seat, try to have it installed a good month before the due date (much better than in the hospital parking lot the morning you drive home). When it comes to the physical installation, even if you read the manual in every language, get it checked at a child seat fitting station. Considering that roughly 80 percent of child safety seats are *not* installed properly, installing it early will give you time to get it checked out. You can find fitting locations via the National Highway Traffic Safety Administration (NHTSA) website www.nhtsa.dot.gov. Select the "Locate a Child Seat Fitting Station" box on the left-hand side of the page, and it will direct you. You can also call your local fire department or police station and ask where to find a child seat fitting station.

When it comes to cost, look for sales but get a good seat. You won't need a convertible seat for several months, so try and find a bargain. Never buy a used car seat or a seat with a history that can't be verified. (You don't want a seat that's been in a car accident, as seats in serious car accidents should be discarded.) When it

CAR SEAT ESSENTIALS:

Install the car seat early and practice before getting to the hospital.

Get it checked at a child seat fitting station (www.nhtsa.dot.gov).

Look for sales during the months leading up to the due date.

Register your seat with the manufacturer.

If your seat is in a serious car accident, replace it.

The life span of a car seat is five years (then replace it).

CAR SEAT SUGGESTION:

Check your car owner's manual and see if you have a LATCH system. Most newer cars have one (it just makes it easier to install the seat or the base). Having a LATCH system means that instead of using the seatbelts in the car, you're able to use the latches and belts on the actual car seat. It's a lot easier and faster.

comes to cutting costs, the car seat isn't the place do it. Our infant seat was our most used baby item during the first few months. We took it absolutely everywhere. In the earliest weeks, we even used the infant seat inside the crib. Our daughter slept better on an incline, and the seat was the most comfortable place for her.

When it comes to the styles, makes, and models, look it up in the *Baby Bargains* book (and no, I get no commission for promoting this, it's just an awesome resource). The book covers the high, middle, and lower tiers of the most common brands. The NHTSA website (www.nhtsa.dot.gov) also provides safety information, ease-of-use information, the latest recalls, and other vital information. And when you buy your seat, make sure you register it at the manufacturer's website. (Include your email address when registering so you'll have a better chance of being informed if there's a recall or another issue that comes up.) I think that covers the car seat.

THE BOTTOM LINE:

Most people install a car seat incorrectly. I was so sure I did it right and checked after writing this tip to prove to myself I was smart, but discovered that I never fastened one of the clips (no BS). I fixed it, but I feel terrible about it.

10

PASSING THE TIME

Things to Do During the Second and Third Trimesters

Tip #65
THE BABY'S SEX: To Peek or Not to Peek, That Is the Question

THE TIP:
That one moment of pure surprise will be a memory that will stay with you forever.

THE STORY:
We waited to find out. I think it's the only way to go with the first child. (We don't have a second yet, but we'll probably find out for #2, maybe not if I have any say in the matter.) The true surprise of the moment is

amazing. As a dad you have a front row seat to "the show," and you are the first to know. You then get to tell your wife, one of the only times you will actually know more about your child than she does. And then comes the fun part—going into the waiting room to tell the grandparents. The look on their faces is priceless. At that point you feel like the most important person in the world. A lot of people like to know the sex so they can "set up" everything before the baby comes home, but it's really not an issue. I wouldn't paint the room pink, but a nice light blue or yellow works for either sex. Everything else can wait until after he/she is born. That moment of surprise will stay with me forever.

—AJ, son 18 months

＊ ＊ ＊

You may be able to find out the sex of the baby via ultrasound as early as week 12. We are one of the few couples we know who waited to find out until the baby was born. We had such a good experience the first time around, we're not finding out again until our second is born. (We might even wait a week after this one is born just to keep ourselves in suspense.)

The speculation was a great distraction (but also

Never waited. Always found out. It helps us plan and made it "real-er" somehow. It helps to kind of envision things and makes the wait more bearable (for her anyway).
—Patrick (expecting #6—a girl)

annoying at times). Most of our family and friends swore it was a boy. My wife swore it was a girl. I just swore. I studied the 20-week ultrasound meticulously looking for a penis. I was convinced I saw a penis, but I later discovered the suspected penis was actually a foot (I was so proud of that big foot for months). We were subjected to lunar charts, the needle/ring on the thread test (if the ring swings in a circle, it's a girl; if it moves like a pendulum, it's a boy), and constant questions about her food cravings (as if that would indicate the sex). How my wife was carrying the baby was also the topic of a lot of discussion. The family thought because she was carrying low it had to be a boy (she's not that tall so anything she carries is low).

Shopping for the baby meant picking out both boy clothes and girl clothes—considering that she likes shopping, this just gave her that much more to do. The stores don't make you buy a lot of these things until you need them. She had two boxes waiting for her once the baby was born. When it came to the nursery, we picked a neutral color and used a wallpaper border that matched the bedding. Whatever the sex, we were ready.

The majority of people I know find out. A lot of times they do it to help plan the nursery, anticipate a bris (ceremonial circumcision), pick a name (see Tip #66), have a sense of control, or

We waited for several reasons: (1) We love surprises. (2) We believe in delayed gratification. (3) We thought it was odd when some of our friends found out the sex of their unborn child, named it, and started addressing it as a real person.

—Mike (son 3 months)

FLIP A COIN, BOY OR GIRL?

Medical Methods to Determine Gender: Ultrasound (assuming the baby exposes him- or herself), amniocentesis (for high-risk pregnancies), and CVS testing (for high-risk pregnancies).

Old Wives' Tales to Determine Gender: Baby's heart rate under 140 = boy, over 140 = girl. Carrying low = boy, carrying high = girl. No morning sickness in the first trimester = boy. Right boob bigger than the other = boy,

plan for medical reasons. It's a personal decision that only a couple can make. I think we chose not to find out because my older brother didn't find out—anticipating, speculating, and coming up with names for each sex was entertaining.

Just know that if you want to wait, it's not as big a hassle as some people lead you to believe. If you do wait, some people might pressure you and want to know. It might be family, it might be friends, it might be your pregnant partner—you should stick to what you believe. If a relative pressures you—like a parent—that person needs to back off. Unless there's a compelling reason—like someone is ill, someone is leaving for a military tour, or some other extreme circumstance—this isn't anyone's decision but yours. Give the people around you permission to be upset if you refuse to find out the sex. There are some things in the world that are no one else's business and this is one of those things. You and your partner get to decide.

Now, if you want to know and she doesn't want to know, or she doesn't want to know and you want to know, you have a real problem. Some couples will have one partner find out and not tell the other. Some couples will find out and not tell family or friends (family and friends can get annoyed if you keep them guessing).

Some couples will not find out, but will have the care-giver notify retailers—*Be careful about this!* The last thing you want is to listen to a voice message from a sixteen-year-old part-time clerk explaining that *his* clothes will be ready for you to pick up when you leave the hospital. If you do confide in a vendor, make sure the information is kept secret. Make a deal and put it in writing—if the secret gets out, you get everything for free. (That should soften the blow.)

FLIP A COIN, BOY OR GIRL? (Contd.)

bigger left boob = girl.
Clear urine = girl (bright yellow urine that glows in the dark = you need to drink more water).
Flipping a coin: heads = boy, tails = girl (actually, I just made the coin one up).

THE BOTTOM LINE:

There are so few surprises in life—for us this was one of the best ever.

Tip #66
THE NAME GAME: What to Call Him or Her…

THE TIP:
If you have strong feelings about the name, make suggestions too. Don't just have her come up with names and shoot them all down.

THE STORY:
My husband and I argued a lot over the name. I didn't expect him to care, but he cared very much. I wanted him to make a list of names he liked, and I'd do the same. He preferred to have me make a list and then he would shoot down names I liked. That was a disaster because he shot down every name until about a week before each of our daughters was born. It's the reason we found out the sex early so we could only argue over one set of names. We found a way to be much more efficient at arguing.

—*Carey, daughters 2 months and 24 months*

> We eliminated any name that either one of us could bash.
> —*Cathy (sons 4 months and 3½ years)*

> Do not tell anyone beforehand. People are rude and will tell you some crazy story about someone named that name. For some reason, after the baby is born, they no longer say those things.
> —*Jay (son 22 months)*

* * *

Picking the name is probably one of the biggest decisions a parent can make. The name you choose will impact your child's entire life. A bad name could turn your baby to a life of crime, isolation, and resentment. A good name can lead a child down the path of prosperity, happiness, and endless joy. It's really that big (but not really).

As the expectant father of a first child, you will find that your vote might not have as much power. In the words of one new mom, "For us, my vote was worth two, and his worth one. A veto from me and the name is gone." It's safe to assume that your pregnant partner will likely have the last word. And that word will be the baby's name.

It's hard to argue with this thinking. (You can try to, but it's never a good idea to argue with a pregnant woman.) If your partner took your last name when you got married, the idea that you also get to pick the first name when it already gets your last name makes it a tough sell. You can argue that if the baby is a girl, her last name will be history when she gets married. So, the first name is the only lasting name. While this might be true, you're not the one gaining the weight, tolerating raging hormones, puking, and pushing out a kid from between your legs. If you're lucky, you can get a middle name and naming rights to the second born. If we lived in the 1800s there wouldn't be a question; you would get naming rights to everything. But we live in the 2000s and

This is one area where both partners should have equal say. I know one couple where the husband hates the son's name. The boy is now five and the father still talks about how he hates the name.

—Tracy (son 3 years, daughter 12 months)

men are equal partners (or just one notch slightly below equal). (***NOTE:*** This is NOT true in all cases. Some women are cool with whatever name you will choose.)

Some things to consider when naming:

1. Will the name result in teasing? Visit a class of eighth graders and ask them to try and come up with demeaning or demoralizing nicknames for the name. You can also pick up the book *The Baby Name Wizard: A Magical Method for Finding the Perfect Name for Your Baby* (by Laura Wattenberg). In addition to some cool naming strategies there is a ranking of how easy it is for a kid to be teased with each particular name.

2. How common is the name? Visit the social security website and check out the list of names dating back to 1879 (http://www.ssa.gov/OACT/babynames/). Harlan was the 824th most popular name in 1973 (when I was born).

3. Who do we name the kid after? Some couples of mixed faiths might find their cultures clash when it comes to naming. Some people will use the first letter or name of a deceased relative's name, some will use the first letter or name of a living relative, some will use the whole name, some the name of a parent, some will

> It's like choosing a restaurant. Give your wife three or four choices that you like and let her pick the winner. Make sure to reject anything you hate right away. Don't waiver.
>
> —*AJ (son 18 months)*

go with junior, II, or III (although it helps if there is a II before having a III).

4. How do we spell it? Consider the name Amy. You can spell it the traditional way, *Amy,* or you can spell it a fancy way: *Aymhee, Aeayme, Aimknee* (silent *kn*), *Aymeeee, Aemhee,* or *Aaamhee.* While all these other spellings prove that you're incredibly clever (maybe not), they can also make life incredibly complicated for your kid. Yes, an interesting name with a spelling that needs to be repeated several times can make for a great conversation piece, but there are other things to talk about. If you do choose an alternative spelling, just make sure you know how to spell it.

TESTING THE NAMES

Naming your child is a personal decision. But still, there will be a time during the name search when you want other people's feedback. Usually, these people are friends and family. Be cautious when vetting names. You'll discover that most people have some association with a name that you love. Your first choice might be the name of an ex-boyfriend who cheated, a sadistic boss who fired someone, a friend doing time for a solicitation conviction, or the name of someone's pet golden retriever or cockatoo. If you love the name, it doesn't matter if anyone else loves it (other than your partner). The name will grow on the people around you. Once the baby is born, the name takes on an entirely different meaning.

NAMING RIGHTS (THE DAY MAY COME):

This hasn't happened yet, but it wouldn't surprise me if someone tried it. Depending on how early you are in the pregnancy, there may be an opportunity to fund your child's future by selling his or her naming rights. Let's say Cheetos wanted to promote their Cheetos Flamin' Hot Crunchy Snack brand. This would make my son's legal name "Cheetos Flamin' Hot Crunchy Cohen." This could be worth millions of dollars in exposure for

If you want feedback, a safe way is to ask the people closest to you to share names starting with the letter you're considering using for a name. For example, if you're using the letter "H," ask if anyone has any "H" names they love or don't love. Listen closely and keep your names a secret. Once you gauge the feedback, you can make your decision privately and tell no one until the birth. Let the world be surprised when they hear it.

PRENATAL NAMES

Now there are some people who will name their baby and refer to the baby by name before he or she is born. I'm not one of those people. If you aren't either, here's a piece of advice: We created a prenatal name for the baby. I'm a big fan of it. You can create ridiculous names that take on personal meaning. Our daughter's prenatal name was "Harle-phanie," a combination between Harlan and Stephanie (like "Brange-lina"). Our current baby's name is "Happy HaHa." I like the name Happy, but we can't name a kid Happy because Happy is too hard a name to live up to. So, we went with it for a prenatal name so we have something to call the baby before it's born. If you have a name and want to keep it a secret, feel free to use any of my prenatal names…or you can always just go with Brangelina.

THE BOTTOM LINE:

The only rule is that you need to figure it out by the time you leave the hospital (or not). Once you see the kid, you'll know the name. If you can't think of a name, just go with Prince—in honor of Prince (the singer).

NAMING RIGHTS (THE DAY MAY COME): (Contd.)

Cheetos over my son's lifetime. And if Cheetos Flamin' Hot Crunchy Cohen were to run for student council, become a star athlete, or end up on TV, radio, or in print…we're talking huge dollars.

Tip #67
HANGING OUT WITH HER BELLY: Talking, Singing, Touching, Petting, Patting, Painting, and Listening to It

THE TIP:
Take pictures—lots of pictures.

THE STORY:
One of the funniest moments of the pregnancy had to be when I was at about 28 weeks along. My hubby would not stop staring at my tummy. Even though he sees me every day, he claims my tummy became ginormous over night. He then grabbed the camera and took pictures of it from every angle…I thought it was hilarious because he was behaving as if he just found out I was pregnant. I didn't mind that he used the word *ginormous* because he was so cute about it. He was 100 percent fascinated. I guess it really sunk in at that moment.

—Amanda, daughters 6 months and 3 years

✳ ✳ ✳

The pregnant woman's belly is one of the wonders of the

> I currently sing to the baby twice a week. I put on a ten- to fifteen-minute concert. My best song is "Nose, Nose, Jolly Red Nose."
>
> *—Jeff (26 weeks pregnant)*

> When he rubs my belly it reassures me that he likes me. I know he loves me. It is the fact that he is touching *me* that makes me feel happy.
>
> *—Nancy (15 weeks pregnant)*

world. If you think she's big now, wait until she's about to give birth. It will look as if she consumed an entire keg on her own in under an hour. It's huge (in a beautiful way). Whatever you do, don't tell her how huge *it* is and poke *it* with your finger. The *it* is attached to her and she will associate these words with how she looks. When in awe, say things like, "You're so pregnant and so beautiful." Always throw in the qualifier after the amazement part.

By the time she arrives in the third trimester, you should be able to feel the baby kick. You'll get a little push, a finger, a toe, a knee, a foot, a hand, and a head. In the early stages she'll feel it before you do. She'll want you to feel it, but you won't be able to feel it. She'll put your hand on her belly and say, "Feel that? Feel it?" And

DOCUMENTING HER BIG BELLY:

Every few weeks or so, take a picture of her belly. Have her stand in the same place and in the same pose and outfit. At the end of the pregnancy, frame some of the photos and give them to her as a gift (a very reasonable push present). You can also have professional pictures taken at a studio of her and her naked belly (it's probably better if you kept yours covered).

I was surprised by just how large her stomach actually got. Hard to believe someone so small can get a belly that big.

—Brad (son 24 months, 22 weeks pregnant)

LISTENING TO HER BELLY:

You can feel it, you can talk to it, and you can just *listen* to it. We used a listening device that she placed just under the naval. There were two pairs of headphones (one for me and one for her). From the moment the monitor is activated you're supposed to hear the magic of your baby's heartbeat in the womb. Beware of these listening devices. While it's supposed to be a magical experience it can be anxiety provoking if you do listen too early in the pregnancy or position the microphone in the wrong place on her belly.

you'll be like, "No." After about forty-five minutes of trying and spasms in your arm from holding it steady, you'll give up trying to feel it. This will go on for weeks. She'll call you over and over again, and all you'll feel is her big belly. Eventually, after weeks of trying, you'll feel something, and it will be the coolest thing ever. Once you feel the baby moving, you'll know she isn't making this whole thing up for attention. She's really pregnant.

At around weeks 27–28, the baby's hearing will be completely developed. This means you can talk to it, sing to it, and do things with it. Keep in mind that you need to talk like the baby has a hearing problem in order to get through the swishing, popping, and whooshing of your partner's stopped-up gassy intestines. Research has proven that babies can identify voices in utero. Speaking to the belly can be a great way to introduce yourself and begin a relationship. Consider playing music, reading books, or just making up stories while chatting with the baby in her belly. Remember, though, that while the baby belongs to you too, her belly is still hers. She might not be into a live concert or storytelling session, so check in and reserve a time to hang out with her belly.

THE BOTTOM LINE:

When you're done having fun and playing with her belly, invite her to have fun and play with yours. It's only polite.

That Magic Marker Line on Her Belly: You might notice a dark line appear from her belly button to her pubic area. It's called the linea nigra and it's a result of the hormonal changes and increased pigment. Some women's are darker than others. This too will slowly disappear over time once the baby is born.

Her Massive Belly Button: As the uterus expands and puts pressure on the navel, her belly button will protrude. Once the baby is born the navel will return to form.

Tip #68
HANGING OUT WITH THE GUYS: Respecting Your Designated Pregnant Driver's Hours

THE TIP:
When she tells you to go out, make sure she really means it.

THE STORY:
My wife and I had a very active social life before she got pregnant. While she was pregnant, she couldn't go out like she used to. One night in particular, she told me to go out and have a good time. She hung out with the wife of the guy I went out with. I came back around 3:00 a.m., and she was waiting for me—upset. She couldn't understand how I could stay out so late. She then told me that she really didn't want me to go out, but she didn't realize this when she told me to go out. She was tired and irritated because I left her to entertain someone all night (although they were sleeping when we got back). I explained that I would have stayed home, but I couldn't know what she wanted because she didn't tell me what she wanted. Her problem was that I should

Don't come home drunk out of your mind. It's really annoying and it reminds a woman that her life has drastically changed, but his hasn't.

—*Ashley (daughter 12 months)*

Respect that she may want to go home earlier than you do.

—*Carey*
(daughters 1 month and 2 years)

have chosen to be at home, and if I went out, I should have known to come home earlier. From that point forward, I asked her to tell me what she wanted and not to be mad if she changes her mind after she tells me what she wants. She agreed.

—*Jon, daughter 4 months*

✳ ✳ ✳

Having a social life and having a pregnant partner is a balancing act. It's balancing her need to know that you love her and your need to still have a life independent of her. It's also balancing her need to feel like you're going to be a role model for your baby and your need to get as much partying in before you need to set an example for your baby.

Going out without her isn't like it was before. How late you can stay out, how much you can drink, and what you can and can't do when you come home will not be the same. The more you can spoil her and pay attention to her, the easier it will be for her to encourage you to go out with the guys. Again, it's all about balance.

For example:

- Balancing means taking her out alone more than you go out with the guys on your own. It also means that when you

My wife encouraged me to party as she was happy to be my designated driver during all three of her pregnancies.

—*Matt (daughter 10 years, sons 7 years and 3 years)*

are out with her, ask if she minds before you order a drink. This is a classy move—unless you get to the point where you've had so much to drink that you can't put the words together to ask her for another. Then the balance has shifted the wrong way.

- Balancing means that when she offers to be your designated driver, you use her services and not abuse them. Abuse would be categorized as calling too often, too late, or too drunk to talk. A tired and nauseous pregnant woman doesn't want to pick up you and your drunk, smoky, stinking friends at one in the morning from a club with hot women who look like they're trying to get pregnant. The chances of her thinking this is funny are about as good as the chances of you getting lucky when you get home.

- Balancing means when she encourages you to go out with the guys, do something for her before you leave her alone. Small gestures like making sure she has dinner, a movie, and something to keep her entertained are nice touches.

- Balancing also means not taking advantage of her generosity. If she allows you to have drinks at the baby shower, don't finish them all off when the guests leave. If she lets you go to the baseball game in her third trimester, don't go out after the game until the middle of the night. If she lets you have friends over for New Year's, it means not blasting loud music all night long.

- Balancing means that if you're planning to fly to Vegas for a bachelor party when she's in her 39th week, make it a one-way ticket because she won't be there when you get back from your trip. There's just no way that's cool, man…

THE BOTTOM LINE:
Avoid too much, too late, or too often.

Tip #69
ULTRASOUND FOR KICKS: A Home Movie of Baby Hanging Out in the Womb

THE TIP:
I'm not sure we would have done it to determine the sex, but after having gone through the experience I think an additional ultrasound at a center is a special experience for anyone—especially with your first baby.

THE STORY:
The hospital technician said, "I think I see a bulge, but can't say for sure." That wasn't good enough for us! The baby wasn't cooperating and getting into a good position to determine the sex. So, we scheduled an appointment at a specialty ultrasound center (not in a mall). I did not ask if they were certified technicians, but I think it was explained in the literature they

provided that this was not a medical facility. We chose the package that gave us a twenty-minute session, four printed photos, a DVD (set to music, which ended up being pretty cool), and gender determination. This cost around $100, maybe a little more (they have several packages). When we got there they took us into a comfortable room that had an ultrasound machine and a big projection screen (very cool—we were able to see images much better). It was just like having an ultrasound at the hospital, except once she found a good angle she would switch it to the 3-D or 4-D image and we could see every feature. I thought it would be kind of creepy, but it was pretty cool. She confirmed the baby was a boy, explained what we were seeing (much more than the technician at the hospital did). She was *really* nice and excited for us which made all the difference. The hospital technician was not very warm, which didn't help our experience. Having the DVD recording was great because we were able to show our parents and friends who were interested. The recording was set to lullaby music, very sweet. I would definitely recommend this.

—*Heather, son 2 months*

* * *

Just because your doctor is done giving ultrasounds doesn't mean you can't get some bonus footage. Stores like Fetal Foto and Little Sprouts Imaging offer parents prenatal ultrasounds. For anywhere from $100 on up (less with a coupon), expectant parents can see live-motion color images of their unborn babies. Some services will broadcast the image live on the Internet.

I got a taste of this when the doctor showed us the ultrasound using 3-D/4-D imaging (similar to what is used at these places). What I saw was a bunch of questions. The skin looked bumpy and scary. Shadows looked like weird growths. I was completely unsure of what I was seeing. The only thing that made it comfortable to watch was the doctor telling me not to worry about it.

When it comes to elective ultrasounds, you'll find some people love them and some hate them. The FDA issued the following caution against prenatal portraits: "Ultrasound is a form of energy, and even at low levels, laboratory studies have shown it can produce physical effects in tissue, such as jarring vibrations and a rise in temperature." Although there is no evidence that these physical effects can harm a fetus, the FDA says the fact that these effects exist means that prenatal ultrasounds can't be considered completely innocuous.

Another reason some advise against commercial ultrasounds is that some operators have discovered abnormalities or complications (read the article, "FDA Cautions Against Ultrasound 'Keepsake' Images" at http://www.fda.gov/FDAC/features/2004/104_images.html). There's also the risk of seeing something that you think looks like a problem but isn't a problem.

If you want snapshots, consult your care provider and consider doing it immediately following an appointment with your doctor. You can also inquire about bringing a DVD or video recorder to the medical ultrasound, where you can probably record it for free. If you do opt for the bonus ultrasound, just let your caregiver tell you that everything is *perfect* first, so shadows don't make you crazy.

THE BOTTOM LINE:
The only thing better than home movies are home movies from inside the womb. This will be perfect for the kid's wedding video (you can show it at the rehearsal dinner).

Tip #70
UNSOLICITED ADVICE: The Things Some People Will Share with You

THE TIP:
If someone offers you advice and hands you a video-tape to go along with it, thank them, and hand it back. Tell them to keep any graphic home videos with their own personal collection.

THE STORY:
When we got pregnant with our first, my sister-in-law ran downstairs to get a video for us. It was labeled "family," which I thought was interesting. She said,

"This is a videotape of me giving birth. When you feel comfortable, watch it. It should help answer your questions." We were about five months along when we popped the tape in. The first shot was of my sister-in-law and her husband sitting at a table—she wasn't pregnant or anything. We thought it was the wrong tape… Then there was a flash of static and the screen cut to the moment of truth. The entire screen was 100 percent vagina and the baby's head coming out of it. When I say 100 percent I mean the *entire* screen was vagina. It was vagina and orb. I felt like I was watching an IMAX movie. I had never seen crowning at that point and my first question to my wife was, "What the F*!K is that?" She explained. What I admired was the videography. My brother-in-law stayed with the shot all the way through the pushing. When the baby was coming out, I felt like I was there for the actual birth. The camera cut away just in time to show a rush of fluid gush out, which was more than I could take. My wife was crying because it was such a beautiful moment; I was somewhere between horrified and titillated. When our baby was born, I stayed up by my wife's shoulders and didn't videotape it. I had seen enough.

—*Corey, daughters 2 years and 4 years*

All these people would tell me horror stories about birth, women screaming, bad things happening, and babies getting sick, but none of it ever happened to us.

—*Kevin (daughter 2 years, 28 weeks pregnant)*

* * *

Friends, family, strangers, medical professionals, priests, rabbis, coworkers, bus drivers, and people in stores, elevators, airplanes, and restaurants will offer you advice as though you were asking for it. Some advice will be helpful, some will be absurd, and some will be offensive and even hurtful. People will offer advice on something as personal as an epidural or as benign as their choice of monitors. (I do like the video monitors.) The helpful advice isn't a problem—it's all the other comments that can wear you down. I've learned that the secret is giving the world permission to be annoying, wrong, and stupid (see Tip #16 for a refresher). This approach makes it so much easier to deal with overeager friends, family, and strangers.

Before getting into the annoying unsolicited advice people share, I should mention that the most invaluable advice I received was from friends who went through the experience a couple months before us. Seeing someone who just went through it and getting advice about the hospital, care, and all the minutia that you can't figure out from a birthing class was valuable and comforting. And now, on to the unsolicited annoying advice…

"LIFE IS GOING TO CHANGE…"
Yes, no shit, Zen Buddhist Master. It's not the fact that people say, "Life will change," it's more *how* they say it. They make it seem so ominous and foreboding. And then when you say, "Yeah, I know it's going to change," they say it again, "No, you don't understand,

it's *really* going to change!" And you're like, "Right, I heard you, it's going to change." Then they get all excited, "*No man, you don't hear me. It's* really *going to change*." I'll tell the truth. It will change, but it will change for the better. I'll get to the rest of this in Tip #92 (just after the baby is born). For advice on how to handle the "It's Going to Change Advice Guy," check out The Bottom Line. But don't let anyone freak you out about the change. It takes time to adjust, but once you're there, it's the *very best change*.

"THIS ISN'T HOW WE DID IT..."

You might be doing something differently than your friends, family, or parents. And doing something differently means opening yourself up to criticism. If there's solid research and it's safe, why not try something different? Doing things differently than the way they've always been done doesn't mean doing something wrong—it means there could be another, better way to do something. Don't be surprised when people question you. When they do, don't try to convince them that you've chosen a better path. Trust that they'll see what you see and then say, "I can't believe it, but you were right..." And even if they don't say you're right, you're making your own choices, and that's what it means to be a parent.

"I HEARD THE MOST HORRIBLE STORY..."

People are going to come up to you or partner and tell you stories that you don't want to hear. I'm not going

IT'S OKAY TO QUESTION CONVENTION:

I read a *New York Times* article about infant potty training which explained how in many parts of the world, potty training starts at birth. I read the book *Infant Potty Training*, and decided to try it at six weeks. People thought we were crazy. Even my husband resisted at first. That was until our seven-week-old pooped and peed in the potty. Everyone was shocked that it could work. Then, all of a sudden I wasn't so crazy.

—Stephanie, daughter 20 months, 8 weeks pregnant

to be one of these people because, really, there's no reason for you to be panicked. The majority of people will *not* experience a problem. Even if you do have some kind of problem, there will usually be answers. If you're expecting and someone starts talking to you about a tragedy or complication, tell them you'd rather not hear about it. Most of the time, they have no idea what they're doing and will stop once they realize their mistake.

THE BOTTOM LINE:

If someone tells you life is going to change one more time, respond with, "What do you mean?" Keep saying, "What do you mean?" after each explanation until the guy offering advice passes out from exhaustion trying to explain this to you or jumps out the window in frustration because you don't get it.

Tip #71

PACKING FOR THE TRIP: Everything You Need to Bring for the Both of You

THE TIP:

Make her a music mix and take it with you.

THE STORY:

A friend of ours told us that it was helpful to have music in the delivery room. They brought their iPod with them. When we went on the hospital tour, they also told us to it would be a good idea to bring music. One night, right around week 35, we put together a mix and burned a CD for the labor. It was just a nice night together. We picked out some of his favorites and some of mine. The hospital had a CD player in the room so we didn't need to bring one with us. The music helped me relax. Now, whenever I hear "Good People" by Jack Johnson, my eyes tear up.

—*Mandy, daughter 2 months*

✳ ✳ ✳

Have her show you what you should bring, not what you think you should bring.

—*Scott (daughter 10 months)*

Do *not* over pack. We brought so much extra stuff that we didn't need. You will end up shuttling everything from room to room when you really should be focusing on your wife's comfort.

—*Eric (daughter 20 months)*

Unless you're having this baby in your own bedroom, you're going to need to pack a bag.

I originally wrote this tip highlighting that the *most* important part of packing isn't what you pack, but when you pack, but that's a big lie. Whether you pack three months ahead of time or three minutes ahead of time, it wouldn't matter if you forgot your phone charger, camera, change of underwear, and the car seat. What matters most is that you know what you need to take with you.

That said, it's a good idea to do your packing more than three minutes ahead of time. But if that's not your style, I respect that. It's not mine. If you're doing it at the last second, at least plan on what you'll need to take so you're not scrambling around when she's ready to go to the hospital. Feel free to dog-ear this page if it will help you when you're rushed.

One suggestion that might complicate your last-minute packing plan is bringing clean clothes with you. For example, if you wear hats, make sure you wash the one you take with you. If you live by the rule that denim is clean until someone tells you that it smells— you might want to change your rule. These are the clothes you'll be wearing when you hold your baby for the first time. The baby will be resting on your chest, laying on your lap, and drooling on your clothes. You'll want them to be clean.

Considering that some hospitals were designed before dads were so involved in the process, your needs are not always factored into the floor plan. You might find out that you have nowhere to sleep. Ask the hospital or birthing facility where new dads sleep. You may have to bring an air mattress or your own pillow.

On the next page I've included a list of things to consider taking. Also, check with someone you know who has given birth at the same place. Ask the question, "What do you wish you brought that you needed?" If you don't know someone, you can stop by the facility and ask some dads hanging out there. If you can avoid packing too much stuff, you'll be thrilled when you see all the other stuff you'll accumulate during your visit. If you forget something, you, a friend, or family member can always run out to get it. The most important items are the birth plan, her stuff, and your pregnant partner. Make sure you bring her or you'll have a big problem.

The following are suggestions from new moms and dads. Following these suggestions, I've provided a list of things I think you should bring. If you're in a hurry, you can rip out the page and use it as a checklist when frantically packing.

Things to keep in mind for her:

- Don't take everything on the list from class. I never touched half of it!
- Take some comfy clothes and a baseball hat if you're a hat person.
- Don't forget her makeup, if she wears it.
- Avoid smelly lotions or perfumes (not good if she's trying to breastfeed).

- Pack light—she will be too gross and dirty to wear the cute new pajamas that you bought.
- Bring her own pillow.
- Pack some books or magazines for her to read.
- Take footies, slippers, or warm socks; consider flip-flops for the shower.
- Pack her favorite snacks.
- Bring a bottle of water (you never know).
- Bring ear plugs! (This is the best advice I have ever received.)

For baby:
- Install the car seat (don't forget the car seat!!!).
- Pack a baby outfit for pictures.
- Pack one special outfit for the trip home.

----------- CUT HERE ---------- CUT HERE -----------

HARLAN'S PACKING LIST
__ Directions
__ The birth plan
__ Hospital paperwork/medical records
__ Car seat
__ Pediatrician's information
__ *The Happiest Baby on the Block* book and/or DVD
__ A mini DVD player and charger (if one isn't available at the hospital)

__ DVDs to watch while passing time (her favorite TV shows are perfect)

__ An iPod or CD player or CDs (if the hospital has a player)

__ Snack foods (trail mix, bars, nuts, and her favorites)

__ Toiletries you would take on an overnight trip

__ Bathing suit (in case you help her in the shower and the nurse comes in)

__ Change of clothes for three days and two nights (make sure the clothes are clean)

__ Comfortable shoes (you'll do a lot of standing)

__ A clean hat (if you're a hat person; don't forget to wash it)

__ Email addresses of people to whom you want to send birth updates

__ Laptop computer and power cord

__ Digital camera or video camera, charger, extra memory card, extra tapes

__ Cell phone and cell phone charger

__ Roll of quarters for vending machines

__ Her suitcase and reading materials

__ An extra bag to haul stuff home

__ Disinfectant wipes

__ If packing for her—comfortable clothes, *not* nice underwear, slippers, toiletries, contact solution (if she wears contacts), glasses, and an outfit to go home in

__ This page of the book (or the whole book)

THE BOTTOM LINE:
___ Your pregnant partner

Tip #72
PATERNITY LEAVE: A Paid (or Unpaid) Vacation with Your New Family

THE TIP:
Take at least a week off. If you can take another consecutive week and still get paid, take it.

THE STORY:
When the baby was born I took a week off. And then within the month I took another week. It was our first baby, and it was a little rough—she needed the help. We get two weeks, but not necessarily two consecutive weeks. In an ideal world, if you could take two consecutive weeks, that's great. I don't think many people can take off for two weeks. But I think the first week is necessary. During the second week, there isn't a lot you can do, unless she's struggling with her health or the baby isn't cooperating. A week is enough. Fortunately both of our kids were easy babies. The second week I just hung out. I played golf once. When the kid was

Today was my first day back after the longest stretch I'd been away from work. Throughout the day, my wife emailed me pictures of what they were doing. It was just awesome. It helped ease my transition. It was nice to feel like I was still involved.

—*Chris (son 2 weeks)*

sleeping, I would help around the house, but after you have the second one, the routine is so much easier. By the end of the week, I was ready to get back to my normal life.

—Kevin, daughter 11 months, son 3 years

✳ ✳ ✳

There's paid leave (vacation days, paternity leave, sick days) and then there's unpaid leave. How much time you take is a personal decision. The reality is that not everyone has the luxury of taking time off. But if you do have the option, take advantage of it—make this your vacation and call it a family trip.

Having a baby can be physically and emotionally exhausting for you (and for her). Taking care of a baby after giving birth can also be exhausting (for her and you). Depending on your health insurance provider and the delivery, she may be back home in less than forty-eight hours. If she has a C-section, she'll be in the hospital longer, and her recovery will be longer and harder. Regardless of the ease of the delivery, when she gets home you need to be a coparent. This means that you'll play an equal role as long as you're both home. She might not be able to walk up stairs, pick up the baby, or do some of the basic things. So if you don't have the luxury of taking time off, make sure she has a family member or close friend who can be there during the first week.

Even if everything goes spectacularly smoothly, you're still going to be exhausted the first week, maybe too exhausted to work. If the baby is sleeping in your room, it might wake up crying to feed every couple of hours. If you were to go back to work, getting up for work wouldn't involve getting up because you'd never get to sleep. Regardless of who is the primary caregiver, it can take a good week to develop a routine and get comfortable with the baby. Until you've worked out the routine, leaving her alone or her leaving you alone can be too much. Besides, during the first week someone needs to be around to run out for diaper cream, a different kind of bottle, dinner, and groceries. She will need you.

Another reason to take time off is that there is always a chance that something won't go as smoothly as you had hoped. In case that happens, make sure you can be there. If you can set aside two weeks, that's even better. You might find out that your benefits include a week or two or three of paid leave—maybe even longer. If you don't have benefits that will pay you for paternity leave, you might qualify for unpaid leave. Under the Family and Medical Leave Act (FMLA), if you work at a large office (fifty or more employees within a 75-mile radius) and you've worked for your employer for at least 12 months and for at least 1,250 hours during the previous year (which comes out to 25 hours per week for 50 weeks), you might be protected under the law. There are some exceptions, but you can check it out by visiting the U.S. Department of Labor's website: www.dol.gov. The best advice is to check with your human resources department and review your benefits.

THE BOTTOM LINE:
This time together is priceless. Take as much as you can afford.

If your place of employment doesn't have paid leave for men and does have paid leave for women, there's nothing wrong with making some noise. Corporate culture is beginning to recognize the role of men, but it's still a slow go. Check out a video by a friend of mine who decided to take matters in his own hands: www.DadsPregnant.com

11

LABOR AND DELIVERY PREP TIME

Things to Help Prepare You for Labor and Delivery

Tip #73
THE BIRTH PLAN: How It Will All Go Down…

THE TIP:
I wish we had planned better for our first.

THE STORY:
When I was in labor, I was unable to speak for myself. I was so self-absorbed (in the labor process) that I couldn't think about much else, let alone articulate my thoughts to the medical personnel. I wish I had known during my first labor how things would go so we could have prepared better. We would have reviewed exactly

what my preferences were and how he would address certain issues with the nurses and doctors. The second time around, we went over exactly what we wanted, and it was a far more comfortable experience and so much better.

—Lesha, sons 7 months and 3 ½ years

* * *

The average man's birth plan:
- Go to the hospital.
- Cheer her on as she pushes.
- Take pictures and videos.
- Celebrate and sleep.

I should be honest—we never wrote down a birth plan. I didn't know to write one (I can write). I never knew to think about it.

Based on the all-day birthing class, the doctor's visits, talking about the delivery, and her plan to nurse, I had a good idea of what she wanted. Fortunately, nothing too crazy happened. Other than her doctor not being able to attend the delivery (he was at his kid's birthday party), we didn't have a lot of unexpected surprises and weren't forced to make a lot of decisions on the fly. Had something unexpected happened (and it happens all the time) or had this been a high-risk pregnancy and she wasn't in a place to answer questions, it would have been my call to execute the birth plan. If she were unavailable to answer questions about the delivery, I would be left to use my best judgment—and using my own judgment during delivery is a frightening prospect.

What's nice about writing down your plan and discussing it in advance is that you can refer to it during the delivery. You can also share it with the team that will be assisting the labor and delivery. Look at the birth plan as if you're an event coordinator and this is your big event. Beyond getting the information to the right people, it's nice to talk through it so you can run the game plan in your head ahead of time. Having a plan can relieve some of the stress that comes with facing the unknown during this experience.

Make sure you talk about this plan early in the third trimester. You never know when the baby will arrive. Here are things to discuss with your pregnant partner and your caregiver before entering the birthing arena:

- Where you will be having this baby (hospital, birthing center, home)?
- When should you go to the birthing location?
- If your doctor isn't available, who will be the doctor doing the delivery?
- Do you have any preferences regarding the birthing environment (music, lighting, etc.)?
- What kind of snacks and other things should you bring?
- Who will be allowed in the delivery room?
- What are the facility's postpartum visiting hours and rules?

- Does she want pain medication? If so, what kind and when?
- Does she want Pitocin? (This helps get the contractions going.)
- Does she want a mirror to assist in pushing? (This helps some women stay motivated.)
- Where does she want you to stand?
- Under which circumstances is an episiotomy performed? (An episiotomy is a procedure in which the area between the birth canal and the anus is cut.)
- Does she want to be mobile or in bed? Preferred position for pushing?
- Does she want a birthing ball? Back massage should back labor start?
- What will your role be in the labor and delivery?
- Do you want to cut the umbilical cord?
- If having a C-section, what is the procedure? Are you allowed in the room?
- If having a C-section, will she hold the baby immediately following delivery?
- Once the baby is born, what's the procedure? Do you have any preferences?
- Will she breastfeed or formula feed?
- Does the facility have a lactation consultant?
- What are you doing with the cord blood?
- Will the baby sleep in the room with you or in the nursery?
- Have you already chosen a pediatrician?
- Do you have email addresses and phone numbers so you can spread the news?

- Who will be point person on the outside to share news and info?
- Do you have a car seat in the car ready to take the baby home?

THE BOTTOM LINE:
If you're reading this on the way to the hospital, you can tear out this page and write some of the answers down. Or you can ask your partner these questions in between contractions during early labor.

Tip #74
THE BIRTH CLASS: The Final Exam Will Be Here before You Know It

THE TIP:
When attending your first relaxation class, make sure you are helping your wife to relax, not focusing on yourself.

THE STORY:
When we attended our first Lamaze-type class, the instructor went through a demo on how to give a massage. After going through the specifics, he told us that one of us should massage the other one. I had my wife go to work on my shoulders. It had been a long day, and I was feeling sore. We looked around the class and every other husband was rubbing his pregnant wife's

shoulders. I was the only selfish asshole in the room getting a rubdown. We quickly switched positions.

—Matt, daughter 10 years, sons 7 years and 3 years

* * *

Welcome back to the classroom.

The birth class is a rite of passage that every expectant father should be required to experience at least once. There's just no good reason *not* to go. Even the longest, most boring, and poorly-instructed class has value. But really, some of them can be interesting, fast-paced, and entertaining. It's like attending a high school class or college class—just being there enables you to absorb the material. If you're assisting in a natural birth (no pain medication and minimal intervention), you'll need to be more familiar with and more involved during all stages of labor. Attending a birthing class will be essential. Regardless of your partner's birth plan, the class will help you, and it will help her to have you there. The more familiar you are with what to expect, the easier it will be for you to remain calm and offer support.

We went to several classes, including infant CPR, Lamaze, and breastfeeding. All were interesting but could have been cut down by about a third as many hours.

—Mike (son 3 months)

Since my wife planned on having a medicated delivery, my role was more of support rather than coaching. We attended two classes. One lasted about eight hours on a

Saturday. The other was an infant CPR class (*very* helpful, especially the infant choking demo). During the all-day birth class, we learned about the three stages of labor (more in Tip #84), pain management, contractions (telling fake ones from real ones), and some breathing and massaging techniques. We were introduced to the fetal monitors. We talked as a group about what excited us about the baby. We changed diapers. We watched videos that were less graphic than I expected. We also participated in a grab bag that included items that patients will encounter during the birth process. I was lucky enough to grab a super-absorbent maxi pad used to soak up the blood and draining liquid (lucky me). Someone else got pregnant woman underwear—what she wears after delivery. (They will not turn you on.)

The most valuable part of the class for me was the hospital tour. Seeing the labor and delivery room, the fetal monitors, and the areas where the baby is examined and cleaned up gave me a clear picture of what to expect. Men are visual creatures—seeing things and being there helps us get a better feel for what's to come. If you can't make it to a class because of work or some other reason, at the very least get a tour of the labor and delivery rooms. Seeing where it will happen will give you a mental picture to help fill in some of the unknowns.

CLASSROOM COURTESY:

Turn off your cell phone during class—no texting, getting scores, or doing anything other than being in class and with your partner.

BONUS CLASS: TAKE INFANT CPR

My wife made me take an additional infant CPR class that included how to help a choking infant. She also required the grandparents and baby-sitter to attend. None of us wanted to go, but it was the *best* and most valuable thing. Take it. In the meantime, you can view an instructional video of infant CPR and a choking demonstration online at http://depts.washington.edu/learncpr/. For information on infant CPR classes, contact your local hospital or American Red Cross (www.redcross.org).

THE BOTTOM LINE:

Whether you go to class or not, the final exam will be on or around week 40. Even if you skipped class, do not miss the final exam.

Tip #75
THE LABOR PARTNER: Helping Her Breath, Push, and Relax

THE TIP:
It takes real engagement from the husband/partner to do it. The more I knew, the easier it was to be there for her.

THE STORY:
We followed the Bradley Method. My role was clear: to help my partner relax—that's at the heart of it. There's lots of prep time involved. We started taking classes in the fourth or fifth month. There's usually a series of twelve classes, but we did a four-course program. We practiced relaxation techniques at home. One exercise involved having her lie in bed and hold ice cubes in her hands. The idea was to practice relaxing her body while holding the ice. We probably did that five to ten times. We must have practiced other relaxation techniques at least twenty times. We would sink into the bed and find the least painful posture that strained the fewest muscles. She also practiced the birthing position on her side. Laying in certain positions

I remember them telling us in class that birth can be exhausting. We need to take breaks when she takes breaks. We need to sit down when we can. We need to eat and stay hydrated. We need to do all these things so when it matters, we'll be fresh.

—Chris (son 20 months)

that allow her to go deep into the contractions is part of it. What was most helpful to me was that being so involved helped me understand exactly what was going on during the birth. I used to think childbirth was painful because a woman is pushing a giant thing through a small hole. Really, it's the contractions that are painful. The Bradley Method explained how the muscles were working to open up the cervix. Labor wasn't just random pain. There was purpose. It's wonderfully empowering for us to have done this together and for me to be able to help her.

—Peter, son 18 months

* * *

I panicked a couple weeks before the delivery because I realized I had no idea what the hell I was supposed to do during labor. Never having been through this before, I didn't know how the sport of giving birth played out. And really, a coach who doesn't know the sport is not a very good coach.

I asked a couple guys who had just been through this if they had to do a lot of "coaching." They too had partners who opted for an epidural so we had similar birth plans. They told me that the doctor and nurses helped them figure it out. They told

She just wanted to be left alone. My job for the first was to make sure there was a mirror there. My job for the second was to hold the camera, the camcorder, and her leg and to make sure the mirror was angled right for her.

—Jim (daughter 2 months, son 3¼ years)

me not to worry. And they were right. The medical team did the coaching. I did a lot of hand holding, counting contractions, watching the fetal monitor, encouraging, and helping her relax between contractions. You catch on quickly. I followed the nurse's lead, and it all unfolded. You enter the birth zone. I'm excited for the next time I get to be there. Having written this book, I feel so much better prepared to be a partner and a coach (if she needs some coaching).

If your partner is having a natural birth, you'll have a bigger coaching role. And if you've gone through the twelve-week Bradley Method program, you'll be well-prepared. You know how things should work. You'll have a birth plan in place. You

QUESTION: The most helpful thing he did for you during delivery?:

ANSWERS:
- He coached, supported, put cool rags to my head, and massaged me.
- He brought me ice chips and encouraged me.
- He held my hand during transition labor, which is the worst.
- Nothing. The poor guy didn't know what to do.
- He stayed calm.
- He turned off the football game.
- He kept telling me that I was doing great.

know the plays. You will have practiced positions. You'll be ready for the main event.

Whether you call yourself a coach or a partner, it helps to know what's going on. Since we're the first

- He stayed by my side the whole time.
- He was patient.
- He listened to what I needed.
- He timed the contractions.
- He massaged my back during back labor.
- He got the nurse and doctor when I asked.
- He made sure the birth plan was followed.
- He didn't argue with me.
- He told me I was strong.
- He was so amazing and attentive to me.
- He looked me in the eyes and kept me calm during my four hours of pushing.

generation of fathers in the delivery room, it's not like our dads can tell us what to do. So, the best thing to do is to ask her. Every woman is unique. One woman will like to be massaged; another wants to be left alone. Some want music, others silence. Some will scream; others will push with quiet intensity. Some will want a cold towel; others will want nothing against their forehead. You'll figure it out.

Being a partner or coach means knowing what's happening and knowing what to expect. The more comfortable you can be with the uncomfortable part of labor, the easier it will be for you to remain calm and focused, which will ultimately help her stay calm and focused. I hope the rest of this book will help you become comfortable in the role you play.

THE BOTTOM LINE:

Attention Coaches (and Labor Partners): Doping *is* legal in this sport.

Methods of Delivery

The History of Lamaze

Lamaze is a philosophy of giving birth developed by Dr. Ferdinand Lamaze in 1951. The goal of Lamaze classes is to increase women's confidence in their ability to give birth. Lamaze classes teach women simple coping strategies for labor, including focused breathing. But Lamaze also teaches that breathing techniques are just one of the many things that help women in labor. Movement, positioning, labor support, massage, relaxation, hydrotherapy, and the use of heat and cold are some others. The Lamaze philosophy of birth is at the centerpiece of Lamaze education, which teaches the following: 1. Birth is normal, natural, and healthy. 2. The experience of birth profoundly affects women and their families. 3. Women's inner wisdom guides them through birth. 4. Women's confidence and ability to give birth is either enhanced or diminished by the care provider and place of birth. 5. Women have the right to give birth free from routine medical interventions. 6. Birth can safely take place in homes, birth centers, and hospitals. 7. Childbirth education empowers women to make informed choices in health care, to assume responsibility for their health, and to trust their inner wisdom. (Source: www.Lamaze.org)

The Bradley Method

In the late 1940s, Dr. Robert Bradley developed a method that embraced childbirth as a natural process that can be managed without pain medication and routine intervention. The Bradley Method is a twelve-week program that focuses on relaxation and pain management through natural means. Bradley believed that it takes months to prepare mentally, physically, and emotionally for childbirth. Bradley classes cover nutrition, exercise, approaches to improve comfort during pregnancy, the role of the coach, introductory information about labor and birth, advanced techniques for labor and birth, complications, C-sections, postpartum care, breastfeeding, and caring for the newborn baby.

Tip #76
WORKING THE DOOR: It's Like Being the Bouncer at Club Push

THE TIP:
Talk about who will be in the room ahead of time. Set boundaries early and avoid hurt feelings later.

THE STORY:
My wife and I talked about what would happen if things got difficult in the delivery room. She had gestational diabetes so she was induced on her due date.

The contractions were very slow at first and her mom was in the room with us for the first six hours, just passing time. As things started to get intense, I started to feel uncomfortable. Her mom was sitting in the chair and not participating. I should mention that my wife wanted a natural delivery (with no medication), and her mom had expressed feelings of not understanding why anyone would want to experience pain. It was my decision to ask her to step out of the room. I told her that my wife would appreciate the privacy. She got a little defensive and wanted to ask my wife if she shared the same sentiment. My wife said the same thing, and her mom walked out in a huff. I walked into the waiting area and explained to her that I didn't mean to hurt her feelings. It wasn't a personal attack on her. There's a lot of emotion and pain involved and I wanted to be respectful. She left the hospital and went home to clear her head. When she came back, my wife had gotten the epidural and things calmed down. We invited her mother back in the room for short periods of time, but she was much better when asked to leave now that we had established boundaries. It all worked out in the end.

—*Lawrence, daughter 17 months*

It never occurred to me that anyone else would be in the delivery room with us. My mother-in-law was disappointed when we informed her that she wouldn't be in there.

—*Irl (son 22 months, 28 weeks pregnant)*

✳ ✳ ✳

Not only are we now in the delivery room, we are the ones working the door. We're like bouncers, only instead of trying to get into a club, people are trying to catch a peek at our partner's BV (see Tip 9: Your First GUYne Exam for an explanation).

Assuming you get a room, you're going to have to monitor who else can be in the room during labor and delivery. Actually it's more like this—unless you're the one who is going to be naked from the waist down, your partner will have the final say about who stays and who goes (and really, being naked from the waist down as an act of support isn't supportive, it's just creepy). Who gets access to the delivery room is her call (although, if she wants ex-boyfriends in attendance, that's crossing the line). You and your partner should discuss this when going over the birth plan (*before* she gives birth—it's not a conversation to have in the midst of labor).

If any of her choices make you uncomfortable or if you think the people affected by her choices will be uncomfortable, talk to them ahead of time. Set boundaries and make sure friends and family have reasonable expectations. If she doesn't want her mom in the room, she can talk to her mom ahead of time. If she doesn't want your parents in the room, you can talk to them about this. And just in case any family or friends who

> She wanted to have a close friend in the delivery room with us. I didn't mind it. I was surprised how helpful it was to have someone else there.
> —Kevin (daughter 2 years, 36 weeks pregnant)

want to be in the room forget that they're not supposed to be in the room, put it in writing and include it in the birth plan in case you need to whip it out. That birth plan can do all the talking for you. If you set the rules early, it shouldn't be a problem.

During my wife's labor, my parents and in-laws were allowed to hang out in the birthing room most of the time. We told them ahead of time that we might ask them to leave at certain times. They were good listeners. When asked to come in, they came. When asked to leave, they left. When asked to roll over, they rolled. When the labor started getting intense, we had to ask them all to leave. And yes, it can be uncomfortable telling your wife's parents to leave—not all parents liked to be asked to leave when their daughter is in the midst of a medical procedure. That's why it helped to have already discussed this in advance.

The last thing you need is to battle a parent in the midst of delivery. If you have an older sibling who has gone through labor and delivery, family members might have similar expectations. Your pregnant partner might not do it the same way. Again, if you talk about this ahead of time, and everyone has the same expectations, you'll have one less thing to worry about the day of the delivery. Should plans change or someone get upset, or should someone start pushing his or her own agenda, bring them back to what this is about—your partner's comfort.

THE BOTTOM LINE:

You are the bouncer. Unlike a bouncer, you shouldn't let hot women inside the room just because they're hot (hot nurses tending to your partner being the exception).

Tip #77
CORD BLOOD BANKING: Saving It Could Mean Saving a Life

THE TIP:

If you have a family history of a disease that is treatable with cord blood, look into cord blood banking.

THE STORY:

We decided to collect the cord blood for our second baby. I'm not sure why we didn't do it the first time—that's a question for my wife. I do know that we decided to do it because my wife has a family history of leukemia, and stem cells might be able to treat something like that. If banking had been around for my wife's relative, there might have been another option for treatment. We were never told about public banking or pressured into private banking. We made our decision based on having a family member with a disease.

—Marc, son 14 months, daughter 4 years

✳ ✳ ✳

Just when you've maxed out the budget, you're going to be asked what you're planning to do with the cord blood. The blood from the umbilical cord is rich with stem cells—the cells that can potentially be used to treat leukemia, other cancers, blood disorders, and a number of other diseases not yet determined. You can choose to do one of three things with the cord blood:

1. Do nothing
2. Store it in a private cord blood bank
3. Donate it to a public cord blood bank

1. DO NOTHING

A lot of people end up doing nothing, but it's only because no one ever mentions that they can do something. For some reason, it's not something brought up by caregivers. I don't know why it's not discussed, but the majority of people I

According to The American Academy of Pediatrics, "the chances of a child needing his or her own cord blood stem cells in the future are estimated to range from one in 1,000 to one in 200,000. Private cord blood banks target parents at an emotionally vulnerable time when the reality is most conditions that might be helped by cord blood stem cells already exist in the infant's cord blood. However, the AAP does recommend private cord blood banking for parents who have an older child with a condition that could potentially benefit from transplantation, such as a genetic immunodeficiency."

We chose to do public cord blood banking so that anyone could have access to the stem cells.
—*Amy (39 weeks pregnant)*

interviewed were either misinformed or not informed of the option to store it.

2. STORE IT IN A PRIVATE CORD BLOOD BANK

When my daughter was born, we chose to do the private cord blood banking because it just seemed like another way to protect our unborn child. We called up the 800 number and spoke to a salesperson. They sent us the collection kit and told us to bring it when we went to the hospital. We informed our doctor several weeks in advance to make sure we were good to go. After the baby was born, the doctor collected the blood and put it in the kit. I called the 800 number and a courier arrived at the hospital and sent it overnight to the storage facility. It was that easy.

While I have no regrets about our decision, I wish there had been more information and better guidance to help us make the decision. With no family history of diseases treated with cord blood, the likelihood of tapping into the banked stem cells is extremely low. There's also no guarantee that the banked cord blood will be effective should a family member ever need to use it.

That said, with medical advancements, it's hard to know which conditions stem cells will be able to help cure in the future. Private cord blood banking will run you anywhere from $1,000 to $2,000, and then there's an annual fee of approximately $100+ a year (look into coupons). When investigating your options, make sure you know how the blood will be collected (usually you'll need to bring a collection kit to the hospital), the costs involved (check to see if the private or public bank will cover the doctor's fees for collection), if you can transfer the cells from one bank to another bank, and what happens if the company goes out of business.

3. DONATE IT TO A PUBLIC CORD BLOOD BANK

Public banking is free and something everyone should investigate (ask your caregiver or contact the hospital where you'll be delivering) When you donate to a public cord blood bank, the stem cells collected become available to anyone who might need them. This means that should you ever need your stem cells, they might not be available. Still, according to the research available, there's a reasonable chance you'll find a match in a public bank.

Donating cord blood to a public bank is relatively easy—as long as you start looking into it before the 34th week of the pregnancy and talk to your doctor or midwife. You can visit the National Marrow Program website (www.marrow.org) for more information. The National Marrow Donor Registry provides patients with "access to more than 11 million donors and cord blood units around the world." When you visit the website, you'll find information that walks you through how and where to donate. You can also contact them in the United States toll-free: (800) MARROW2 (1-800-627-7692). Outside the United

States, call (612) 627-5800 and once connected, dial 0 for the operator.

The collection process for donating to a public cord blood bank is similar to the process when banking privately. The main difference is that once it's collected anyone will have access to your cord blood donation.

THE BOTTOM LINE:
Whether you do it privately or publicly, bank your cord blood. It's too valuable to throw away.

Tip #78
THE PEDIATRICIAN: The Doctor Will See Your Baby Now

THE TIP:
Not all women will interview the doctor.

THE STORY:
As a teacher, I know that nothing can truly prepare you for the classroom—you just have to wait until you're there. That's how I felt about the pediatrician. Nothing I can observe in an interview can show me; it was more about what I saw once the doctor was interacting with my son. I asked all my friends who they had gone to and what they experienced. I asked the parents of students in my class. When we filled out the hospital forms, we had to list a doctor. The doctor I

listed didn't end up being the doctor we used. The original doctor wasn't available to meet my son in the hospital, so another doctor from the practice came in. I had never met her before. We had an instant connection. I was having problems with breastfeeding and she was like my coach. While she wasn't taking on more patients, she made an exception for us. And that's how we found our doctor.

—*Leslie, son 22 months*

* * *

I had no idea that we had to find a doctor for the baby before the baby was born. The thought never entered my mind until my wife entered the thought into my mind by saying, "We need to find a doctor for the baby." It's strange to get a doctor for an unborn child. The paternal instincts hadn't quite kicked in for me at that point. So, finding a doctor meant having to imagine what it would be like to be a father. And that's virtually impossible because until you're a father, you can't know what it feels like to be a father.

When the baby is born, the pediatrician (or family doctor) will come to the hospital or birthing facility and examine the baby. We were required to fill out paperwork during pre-registration and list our pediatrician. So the decision needs to be made

When interviewing your doctor, inquire about circumcision. If you decide to have your child circumcised, will the pediatrician do it, the obstetrician, or a mohel (if having a bris)?

—*Chris (son 2 weeks)*

before the baby is born. A lot of women take the lead on this one (must be the maternal instincts). Had I known a little more about what to ask and what to look for, I probably could have been more supportive, but it was all foreign to me.

Some people interview doctors and some interview their friends to find the best doctor. However you and your partner approach this one, here are some questions that can help you figure out the best fit for your personality. As long as the doctor has a great reputation and is in-network, you'll be in good hands. Once you see the doctor in action with the baby, you'll figure out the rest.

QUESTIONS TO ASK IN ORDER TO FIND THE RIGHT FIT

Doctor's Training
- How long has the doctor been practicing?
- Where did he or she go to school?
- What are his or her particular specialties?

Doctor's Personality
- Why did he or she choose to become a doctor?
- Does he or she have kids of his/her own?
- Favorite part of the job?
- Least favorite part of the job?
- The biggest mistake new parents make?
- The thing new parents do best?

Doctor's Philosophy

- Thoughts about breast-feeding?
- Thoughts about formula feeding?
- Thoughts about immunizations?
- Thoughts about the family bed? (see Tip #97)
- Thoughts regarding circumcision?

Doctor's Office Services

- What are regular office hours?
- Are there weekend hours?
- When are sick appointments scheduled?
- When is well-care scheduled? What is the schedule for newborns?
- Is there a separate waiting area for sick kids (so that well and sick kids aren't intermingled)?
- How long does it take to get an appointment (emergency or non)?

Want to See If Your Doctor's Certified? Visit the American Board of Medical Specialties at www.abms.org.

- Will you always see the same doctor?
- How long are well-care appointments?
- How long are sick-care appointments?
- Does the doctor generally run on time?
- Does the doctor have a specific "phone-in hour" to answer calls?
- How long does it take to get a return call during regular office hours?
- What is the policy regarding after-hours calls? Who calls back? How long does it take to get a call back? Is there a fee?

Paying for Care
- Is the doctor part of your insurance plan?
- Do they accept credit cards?
- Cancellation policy?

Questions for Yourself
- Is the location convenient?
- Is parking easy?
- Is the size of the practice too big for you? Too small?
- What do other parents say?
- Most importantly, do you get a good feeling from the doctor? Is this someone you feel comfortable talking to?

THE BOTTOM LINE:
If she takes the lead on this one, help out by asking coworkers and friends for recommendations.

Tip #79

THE TIP:

When discussing your birth plan with the doctor, the part about the pain medication is her decision.

THE STORY:

It was the "labor talk," and the doctor was asking me what my plan was regarding pain medication. Obviously, for me it was no question. I already knew I was going to have an epidural. When the doctor asked what I planned to do, my husband chimed in and said, "Is it necessary to get an epidural? Because I've had cavities filled without novocaine before." The doctor explained that it's not the same thing. Then my husband continued to describe his experience and question my need for medication. He was totally serious about it too. The doctor explained that he didn't think anyone who's not a woman can know the experience and understand the feelings. I just looked at my husband and said, "You're f*!kin' crazy. I'm getting an epidural." Once the baby was born and he saw me go through twelve hours of contractions before getting to the hospital,

We had to leave the room for about fifteen minutes when they did the epidural. She was looking pretty groggy at the time when I left with her mom. When we came back, she was all perky and high.

—*Chris (son 20 months)*

he realized how stupid he was to say that. I think he was just trying to be a tough guy.

—*Grace, son 2½ years*

✳ ✳ ✳

Until a man can deliver a 7½-pound baby through his penis, this one is her call. If your idea of pain relief and her idea of pain relief don't match up, she wins. When it comes to pain management during labor and delivery, women have strong feelings one way or the other. It's either "Hell Yeah!" or "Hell No!" But it's something that needs to be talked about and included in the birth plan (see the box at the end of this tip for the most common pain management options).

HELL YEAH—GIVE ME THE EPIDURAL

One of the most talked-about forms of pain management is the epidural. The epidural block is administered through a flexible tube inserted into the back near the spinal cord. The procedure takes about twenty minutes. The medication can take up to twenty minutes to kick in. If administered too late, it can be ineffective. My wife was aware of this and made sure she got the epidural early into active labor (no way was she

> I delivered all three of our children totally naturally, and it brought my husband to tears after our first was born. He just kept telling me how incredibly strong I was.
>
> —*Cathy (sons 10 months and 3 years, daughter 4½ years)*

missing the pain med window). Once her contractions started to get painful, she called in the anesthesiologist and asked him to deliver the goods. He was her new best friend.

Here's how our epidural went down. The anesthesiologist asked me to leave the room during the fifteen-minute procedure. Once the meds kicked in, she was so damn happy. While the epidural numbed the pain, she could still feel the pressure of the contractions and the baby passing through the birth canal. (Some women have a harder time feeling the contractions while on medication.)

Of course with any procedure there are risks, but that's something you should discuss with your caregiver and the anesthesiologist. Whatever she chooses, it's helpful for you to have an idea of what you can do to help. This is where birthing classes, breathing, labor positions, back massages, and other techniques come in.

HELL NO—NO PAIN MEDS FOR ME

If your partner is opting for a natural birth, this doesn't mean a vaginal birth. A natural birth actually means a birth with as little medical intervention as possible. In a perfect world, for her this would mean no pain meds, no meds to induce labor, no IV (this can restrict movement), and several other criteria discussed in your birthing class. Basically, her body dictates how labor progresses—not the caregiver. Many women who plan on having a natural birth feel strongly about *not* administering medication. The problem is that never having had a baby, and never having experienced labor, it's hard to know what she will feel and what she will want until she gets there.

Make sure you know what she wants, but let her know that what she wants might change and you support her decision. After thirty-six hours of labor, she might change her mind. After ten minutes she might change her mind. Avoid telling her to suck it up or pressuring her to work through the pain if she wants pain meds. Listen to her. If you're unsure if she's just complaining or not saying what she really feels, create a signal ahead of time that will indicate to you that she *really* wants meds. It can be some kind of code like, "*Medicate me, you bitch!*" Or it can be a hand gesture, like waving her middle fingers on both hands in concentric circles. It can be a physical action, like slapping your cheek. Or it can simply be, "Pain medication please." If she has a doula or a midwife, make sure she knows the birth plan. Having it in writing helps clear up any confusion.

Whatever happens, support her decision. The *most* important thing is that the baby is healthy and that mom is healthy. The problem is that women who want a natural delivery and change their plan mid-labor have been known to feel a deep sense of guilt. A healthy baby is nothing to feel guilty about. Changing her plan should be part of the plan.

THE BOTTOM LINE:

The truth is that it really doesn't hurt (they're just being dramatic). And NO, I'm not serious. If you believe that, you're in deep trouble.

Pain Management Options

(Source: womenshealth.gov)

Epidural Anesthesia

A doctor injects medicine into the lower part of the backbone or spine. The medicine blocks pain in the parts of the body below the shot. During a contraction, the feeling of pain travels from the uterus to the brain along nerves in the backbone. Epidurals block the pain of contractions by numbing these nerves. Epidurals allow most women to be awake and alert with very little pain. Many women who get epidurals do not feel any pain during contractions. Medicines used in epidurals include novocaine-like drugs that block the pain in that region combined with opioids like fentanyl.

Some disadvantages of an epidural include the following:

- It can make her shiver.
- It can lower her blood pressure.
- It can make her feel very itchy.
- It can cause headaches.
- It may not numb the entire painful area, so some women continue to feel pain in the abdomen and back.

Intravenous or Intramuscular Analgesic

Pain medicine is administered through a tube inserted in a vein (intravenous) or by injecting the medicine into a muscle (intramuscular). These medicines go into the blood and help ease the pain. Opioids including morphine, fentanyl, and nalbuphine are usually used for this type of pain relief. This option does not get rid of all the pain. Instead it usually just makes the pain bearable. After getting this kind of pain relief, a woman can still get an epidural or spinal pain relief later.

Some disadvantages of getting intravenous or intramuscular analgesics include the following:

- They make her feel sleepy and drowsy.
- They can cause nausea and vomiting.
- They can make her feel very itchy.
- These medicines cross into the baby's bloodstream and can affect the baby's breathing and heart rate and cause him/her to be very sleepy after birth.

Pudendal Block

A doctor injects numbing medicine into the vagina and a nearby nerve called the pudendal nerve. This nerve carries sensation to the lower part of the vagina and vulva. This is only used late in labor, usually right before the baby's head comes out. With a pudendal block, she has some pain relief but remains awake, alert, and able to push the baby out. The baby is not affected by this medicine, and it has very few disadvantages.

Spinal Anesthesia

A doctor injects a medicine into the lower part of the backbone. This medicine numbs the body below where the medicine was injected. Spinal anesthesia gives immediate pain relief, so it is often used for women who need an emergency C-section. Spinal anesthesia uses numbing medicines similar to novocaine combined with opioids like fentanyl.

Some disadvantages of spinal anesthesia include the following:

- It numbs the body from the chest down to the feet.
- It makes her feel short of breath.
- It can lower her blood pressure.
- It can cause headaches.

Tip #80
YOU RUN THE SHOW: You Are Her Eyes, Ears, and Voice

THE TIP:

If something doesn't feel right, let someone know. Don't let anyone else run the show. You need to do what you feel is right.

THE STORY:

The labor and delivery went along as well as could have been planned. I wasn't concerned, but the nurse and the doctor said the placenta was very large. Once the labor and delivery was complete, the nurse felt my wife's abdomen during recovery. She said it felt like her bladder was full and asked her to go to the bathroom. In hindsight, this seemed unusual because she had a catheter which had emptied the bladder. There was a good amount of blood, but no one thought that was unusual because the catheter had just been removed, and blood is part of labor and delivery. Again, in hindsight, I would have asked the doctor to feel if the uterus was contracting properly. About an hour or two later, we moved from the labor and delivery room into the hospital room. When the nurse felt my wife's abdomen, she noticed that my wife was bleeding and had soaked through a pad. The nurse changed the pad which started soaking through again. That's when I told her to call the doctor. She wanted to wait and see how things progressed. I insisted that we should call the doctor. She then called the chief resident. When the resident arrived, she noticed there was a lot of hemorrhaging. Everything moved very fast, but a hemorrhage cart was brought into the room, and there was a lot of blood. They scraped out the uterus so that the uterus could contract and stop bleeding. She was lucky enough not to need blood.

—*Mike, son 9 months, daughters 5 years and 7 years*

✳ ✳ ✳

If the birth plan is the blueprint for the job, you're the foreman. You are the one to make sure that everything goes according to plan (the birth plan). Given that your partner will be busy during labor, you're going to be her eyes, ears, and voice. Even if a doula is assisting, you still need to be involved in the process.

It's hard to be in charge when so much of this is new and unfamiliar. This is the reason why birthing classes, conversations with other guys who have been there, and a book like this can be helpful.

One thing about being an advocate: It can be uncomfortable at times. Not everyone will be patient with you. Someone might snap. Someone might get nasty. Not everyone will respond to you the way you want them to respond. Not all caregivers will mesh with you. At the same time, the majority of the medical team will be

Be friendly during shift changes.

Know where the nurse's station is.

Know how to page for help.

Be kind and courteous when meeting the team.

Show everyone the birth plan (write it out).

Listen to your partner when she needs something.

Listen to your instincts when you need something.

If you have questions, always ask them.

If you don't get an answer, ask again.

July is the season for new residents—ask to speak to an attending physician.

happy to address your and your partner's needs.

One way to get the medical support team on your side is to acknowledge them when you meet them. Introduce yourself. Ask how they're doing. Stop for one second and let them know how much you appreciate them. Explain that you're a first-time father. Let them know that you might have questions and that you appreciate their patience. Start a relationship with them. Share the birth plan with them (another reason why having it in writing is useful). They will be the most important people during the birth—second to your pregnant partner. Share snacks with them. Offer them a drink when you run down to the cafeteria (not a scotch, a Diet Coke). Show them that you appreciate and value their time and services. Give 'em a little love—that's it.

Appreciate that shifts will change and, most likely, the nurses you meet when you are admitted will not be the same nurses who are there when your baby arrives. Whenever there is a shift change, make an effort to be as nice as you were the first time around. This can get hard as you get tired and the labor intensifies, but as an advocate, you need to do whatever you can to have a relationship with the people who will be in charge of her care. Share your birth plan with whoever takes over.

NOT EVERYONE WILL RESPOND

Most medical professionals do *not* make mistakes, but some do. When you play the role of a vocal, caring, and educated partner, it means asking questions which in turn means requiring attention—not all caregivers want to be asked questions or want

PREGNANCY Q & A:

QUESTION: Most helpful thing your man did during delivery? ANSWER: This was our second child and he's a surgery resident. The anesthesiologist didn't arrive until 45 minutes after I asked for medication—I desperately needed the epidural. My husband found the guy and told him, "That's my wife in there and if you don't come and give her that shot, I will."

—*Cathy (sons 4 months, 3½ years)*

to give you attention. *Never* hold back from asking questions. When a nurse comes in and injects something into your partner or baby, ask what's being injected before the liquid flows. If the fetal monitor seems to be out of position or you're unsure of what the lines mean, ask. If the heartbeat seems too fast or too slow, say something. If something is beeping, page a nurse and ask. Ask them to double-check dosages when administering medication to your partner or the baby. When the doctor checks her cervix to determine her progress, ask him what's happening and to explain if you don't understand. As an advocate, you have a right to know.

THE BOTTOM LINE:
Kiss up to the nurses, but don't kiss them (not cool while your partner is giving birth).

Tip #81
GETTING IT TO COME OUT!: Walking It Out and Sexing It Out

THE TIP:
Even "Dance Dance Revolution" on the Wii won't get it out.

THE STORY:
Today is my due date and I've been trying to meet my baby for the past two weeks. I've made a point to walk to the train every day during my commute. When I get to work I'm upright and active. Last week I had a prenatal massage by someone trained in acupressure. She

worked the pressure points in my ankles and feet for a good hour, but it didn't work. This past weekend, a friend of ours got the Wii. We played "Dance Dance Revolution" for a good hour. When that didn't work, I played Wii tennis for a half hour. It didn't hold my attention. We walked around the malls a couple of times and still nothing. I've continued taking my prenatal yoga classes (that's supposed to help). Today I cooked a lot, thinking that being upright would help. All I have is a freezer packed full of food, but still no baby. I'm coming to terms with the fact that I have no control. I have to be patient and wait it out. The anticipation is so hard.

—Amy, 40 weeks pregnant

* * *

There will be a point when she wants it out. She will be done—like when the red popper sticks out of the turkey. She will run out of patience. She will be unable to sleep, unable to hold her pee, and she will be all-around completely 100 percent done. Even the happiest pregnant women will sour when their due dates have come and gone and the pounds keep packing on.

Lots of sex didn't work, but trying to "loosen the seal" was fun anyway.
—Patrick (expecting #6)

We tried everything—sex, scrubbing the floor, going for walks (which is healthy anyway so do that), spicy food... *None of it works!*
—Molly (son 4 months)

How labor begins is something that science hasn't quite figured out. We have been able to create a drug that can start contractions and induce labor, but we don't know how to make it happen naturally. Other than a C-section or induction, it's just a waiting game.

Over the years, pregnant women have tried a number of things to get it out of them—having sex, walking for hours, exercising, stimulating the nipples, eating spicy foods, eating pineapple, applying pressure to the ankles, acupuncture, and fasting are only some of the old wives' tales you'll hear about (interesting how they're never "young wives' tales").

Talking the baby out, walking it out, and sexing it out are some of the techniques I would suggest. Should your doctor give you the okay to have sex during the final days of the pregnancy (not all of you will get the green light), go at it. It is said that semen has a similar make-up to the chemical that can trigger labor (it's science, not BS). When she suspects you of trying to trick her into having sex with you, read this paragraph to her. If this isn't enough proof, Google "semen-inducing labor." But before you get too excited about having sex, understand that extremely pregnant sex isn't always hot sex. I mean, it's hot if the air conditioning is broken and you're having pregnant sex in Florida in August, but don't

I asked the baby the come out on a Friday so we could have the weekend, and on Friday afternoon she went into labor. He was born Saturday. The baby heard me.

—*Steve (son 9 months)*

expect it to rank in your top ten encounters. Still, any sex you can have before she goes into her sex hibernation is good sex.

WARNING: If she's approaching her due date and has yet to give birth, people will call and ask if she's close. Most of these people will be family and friends who will know when she goes into labor. She's likely to get annoyed with everyone asking her the same question. All she wants to do is *not* think about the fact that she's *not* in labor. Having people call will just be a reminder of what she's trying to forget. You will act as the buffer for these calls. If you get tired of being a buffer, a lighthearted effective way of protecting your pregnant partner is to create a special outgoing voicemail message. You can follow the script I've provided or any variation:

"Hi, this is (insert your name). We're not here right now to take your call. It's not because (insert her name) is in labor, but because we're trying to go into labor. This means we're either walking around a mall or having sex. When we're back from the mall or done having sex, we'll call you back. Thanks!

THE BOTTOM LINE:
The sex induction strategy is not for you, it's for her.

12

THE BIRTH DAY

From Your Door to Delivery Room and Back Again

Tip #82
GOING INTO LABOR: Driving Like a Maniac and
Hoping for a Room

THE TIP:
When she goes into labor, your nesting instincts will
kick in. And that can mean feeling like an idiot.

THE STORY:
Being half-asleep and half in disbelief, I muttered
something unintelligible like "Mhhhwahhh?" She then
told me that she had been using the bathroom when all
of a sudden a gush of liquid came out. And since it was

Make sure you have gas. Make it a rule to never have less than a half tank of gas during the final trimester (a tough thing to do). Women in labor do not like sitting in the car while you pump.

Leave jewelry at home. She might need to take off her jewelry, and it's too easy to lose.

Make sure she leaves valuables at home.

I heard my wife screaming at 7:30 a.m. about water. We had a leaky toilet the night before. So I grabbed a plunger and towels and ran upstairs. She laughed at me and asked how I was going to deliver the baby with that.
—*Jeff (father of two)*

still leaking out of her, either her water had broken or she was having the world's longest "accident." To be honest, until we got to the hospital, it didn't fully hit me that her water had broken. Or if it did, that this meant the baby was going to be delivered. But either way, we needed to get to the hospital, so I sprang into action—which meant acting like an idiot. We didn't have a bag packed yet, so my wife calmly began packing while I got dressed and began pacing back and forth, unsure of what to do with myself. I kept asking her over and over if I should wear a baseball cap, until I realized that I was, for some reason, asking a woman going into labor to focus her attention on whether or not I wore a hat.

—*Peter, son 6 months*

✳ ✳ ✳

The moment she starts going into labor is the moment the man realizes she's actually going to have a baby. Even after nearly 40 weeks of pregnancy, until she starts going into labor, it's not real for us. She's known this for months, but then this thing has been kicking her every day to remind her. Once the moment hits, we realize that she needs to get to the hospital and have this baby.

A man's instincts are to take her to the hospital ASAP. A woman's instincts tend to be to clean herself up—as if she's about to go to senior prom. My wife took a shower, dried her hair, and had a pedicure the day before. I started to get jealous of the doctor—she rarely got so dolled up for me. While she got prepped, I sat there in a state of shock thinking, "Holy shit, I can't believe this is happening." By the time my wife was ready to go, I

Refer to a list of things to do right before leaving— take out garbage, adjust the thermostat, etc. It's hard to think in that moment, so if you have a list you won't have to do any thinking.

CALL YOUR HEALTH INSURANCE PROVIDER.

Many health insurance providers require that you notify them within a specified period of time when she is admitted for delivery.

I was very anxious when she went into labor. Make sure you know the route (especially if you go at night) and exactly where to park if you arrive after hours.

—*Mike (son 12 months)*

SIGNS SHE'S IN LABOR:

Call your doctor or mid-wife if:

- Contractions come at regular and increasingly shorter intervals. Contractions should also become stronger over time and continue even when changing positions.
- She has lower back pain that doesn't go away.
- She feels premenstrual and crampy.
- Her water breaks (can be a large gush or a continuous trickle).

> I almost got into two accidents on the way to the hospital. There was a blizzard and a van almost ran into me. Then I was following a snow plow when it started to back up and just missed me. My wife was yelling at me the whole time.
>
> —Scott (daughter 9 months)

was just starting to put my things together. She had to wait a couple of minutes while I packed and went through my list. Women are allowed to do whatever is on their list, but if you delay them in any way they get pissed off. Women in labor are *not* very patient (a shocking revelation, I know).

Should she go into labor and should she leave you alone to pass the time while she showers and puts on make-up, it's a good idea to go through the "what to pack list." It's also a good idea to have your "going to the hospital outfit" in mind. It sounds ridiculous, but this way you don't have to think about what to wear. It can be hard to think at that moment. You can also put together a list of things you need to do when you leave the house— things like taking out the garbage, lowering the heat or air conditioning, turning off the outdoor lights, unplugging anything that needs to be unplugged—all the same things you would do if you were going out of town for a few days. Writing it down in advance will help you focus.

Once you arrive at the hospital, you're not guaranteed entry. You can get rejected at the door. Unless you have a planned C-section or are being induced, there's no guarantee that they will give you a room. And even if you get a room, there's always a chance they can send you home once the doctor checks her out.

In order to get a room, she needs to be at a certain point in her labor. That point can vary based on your caregiver and how busy the facility is. But there's a reasonable chance you might get rejected. The doctor might tell you to take a walk and come back in a few hours or in a few days. You won't know until you get there.

SIGNS SHE'S IN LABOR: (Contd.)

- She has a bloody (brownish or red-tinged) mucous discharge. This is probably the mucous plug that blocks the cervix. Losing her mucous plug usually means her cervix is dilating (opening up) and effacing (becoming thinner and softer). Labor could start right away or it may still be days away.

(Source: www.4women.gov)

THE BOTTOM LINE:

She can take as much time as she wants when she goes into labor, but the moment you start making her wait, you become an accidental asshole. Women in labor are not very patient.

Tip #83
PASSING THE TIME: Eating, Drinking, Watching the Breastfeeding Channel

THE TIP:

Don't leave the delivery room when she's in labor. If you do, don't go home and clean to pass the time.

THE STORY:

My husband is a cop and one of those testosterone kind of guys. With our first child, it was hard for him to understand that I needed him. He was the type of man who didn't know what to do when I was having contractions. I don't know if it was because he was scared or nervous, but when he saw that I was in so much pain, he said that he had to leave and go clean the house. I was so pissed. I was trying to get through my labor, and he just got up and left. The doctor thought I'd be there all day long, but I had the baby three hours later. When my husband came back, my feet were already in stirrups and I was pushing. The second time around, he's much better. I told him he wasn't leaving this time.

—Maria, daughter 2 years, 34 weeks pregnant

✳ ✳ ✳

Once you get settled into the room, there's a reasonable chance you'll do a lot of sitting, snacking (covertly), and avoiding sleep until the action heats up. It's not all huffing, puffing, and counting contractions. When things pick up, they'll move fast. But before then, it can be a slow crawl. It's like watching a baseball game between two last place teams at the end of September. Labor can be slow—very slow.

If your partner is having a natural delivery with no pain meds, you'll be busy helping her through early labor. If your partner is taking pain medication, you may face hours of sitting and anticipating. It's exhausting to wait—physically and emotionally (but never complain that you are tired). It was hard enough sitting through the thirty-minute video at the birthing class— imagine thirty-two hours. Plan on how you'll pass the time. The following are some things to keep in mind:

My husband kept playing with everything in the delivery room. He was playing with the diapers, the hand sanitizer (he must have applied Purell a hundred times), the umbilical cord scissors, the cabinets—after a while I tuned him out, but when he started playing with the lights I lost it.

—Jodie (son 2 ½ years, daughter 10 months)

THINGS TO KEEP IN MIND WHILE PASSING THE TIME

- **Sleeping during labor:** She might sleep, but you shouldn't sleep—unless she wants you to sleep. If you do sleep, set your cell phone for thirty-minute increments. You want to be awake and aware. You don't want someone to perform a C-section while you're dreaming that she had a C-section.

- **Playing music:** Make sure to take an iPod or some CDs to play. It helps to pass the time. It's also something she'll enjoy focusing on when the labor gets intense. Check ahead of time if the facility has a music player.

- **Eating and drinking:** You need to eat and stay hydrated. Do your eating and drinking outside the room. If the food smells, do it far enough away where she can't smell the fries. Pack non-smelling snacks like energy bars, trail mix, and nuts—even if Cheetos is sponsoring the birth (see Tip #66).

- **Cell phone/texting:** Women in labor don't like it when guys are on their cell phones talking about their fantasy baseball draft. You might be nervous or anxious, but don't sit there talking on the phone. Use it sparingly. If someone calls for her, don't hand her the phone without her okay.

I went through 36 hours of labor. He actually sat down in a chair and fell asleep! I screamed at him to wake up and when he wouldn't I threw a roll of medical tape at him. When that wouldn't wake him up I threw a frozen bottle of water at him. It hit him right in between the eyes!

—Ashley (daughter 12 months)

- **Watching TV and movies:** SportsCenter might be soothing for you, but not for her. If you happen to come across the breastfeeding channel, don't stay on it for too long. If she has a favorite TV show, buy the full-season DVD set and bring it along. You can also bring movies to play on your DVD or computer (again, her choice).
- **Visitors and guests:** While you might not have planned to have friends or family in the delivery room, it's nice to have other people in the mix to spice things up (if she says yes, of course). Just make sure they know that when things start moving, they will have to move back to their waiting room seats.

PREGNANCY Q & A:

QUESTION: Least helpful thing you did during delivery?
ANSWER: Made phone calls to work. To this day she believes that work took precedence.
(Patrick, expecting #6)

ANSWER: He sat around eating Chinese food while I was in pain. (Elizabeth, daughter 7 months)

- **Smoking:** If you step outside for a smoke, don't bring the stink back in with you. That might disgust her. Better yet, if you do smoke, just don't smoke while she's in labor.
- **Don't be funny:** My wife told me that there's no room for joking during the labor. I thought she was joking. It turns out that she was serious. Once the epidural took hold, she appreciated the joking.
- **Seat fillers:** Like having a seat filler at the Academy Awards, if you need a break, get a stand-in. Find a family member to take your place while you run out for a snack or head to the cafeteria.
- **Leaving:** Do not leave her for long periods of time. She will need you there.
- **Working:** Do not bring work to the labor room. She wants your full attention.
- **Expelling gas:** Leave the room when you get the urge. If anything, do a tester in the bathroom to see if your gas smells. If it doesn't smell, then feel free to let it go. Otherwise, be kind and hold it in.

THE BOTTOM LINE:
Things will go from 5 miles per hour to 100 miles per hour. Just don't fall asleep at the wheel.

Tip #84

THE TIP:

It might be fast and easy—easier than anyone anticipated.

THE STORY:

At 8:00 a.m. I thought I was in false labor. At 9:00 a.m. we started timing the contractions. At 10:00 a.m. we called the doctor and were told to go to the hospital. At 10:15 a.m. my water broke. It was kind of a trickle, and then with each contraction, it increased. My husband was driving and timing the contractions. When we got there, they said that today was the day! At 1:30 p.m. they moved me into the delivery room and at 2:15 p.m. I got an epidural. I was really glad—I was having contractions since 8:30 a.m., and the pain was starting to get intense. When I got the epidural, they checked me and said I was 6 cm dilated (they only checked me three times because my water had broken, and they didn't want to risk an infection). They told me to wait until 6:00 p.m. to start pushing because I was strep B positive, so they wanted me to have some medication beforehand. At 6:00 p.m. they said it was time to push.

He came out fourteen minutes later. There was no tearing and no episiotomy; everything went well!

—Kate, son 2 weeks

THE TIP:
It might be long and hard, but it will be worth it.

THE STORY:
We had been at the hospital for several hours before the pushing began—in fact, this was our second time there since we'd come in the night before with a "false alarm." Once the pushing began at about 9:00 p.m., it kept going for three hours. We were getting pretty tired, frustrated, and disappointed by the third hour. Our nurse kept giving us false hope by saying "good push," when in fact there was little progress. It was her way of cheering us on, but we just wanted the truth. After about two and a half hours of pushing and twenty-four hours of labor, we said to each other that we would just do a C-section if that's what it's going to take. My wife was tired, and she was feeling claustrophobic from wearing an oxygen mask. It wasn't ideal but seemed at the time to be a better scenario than pushing for another thirty minutes with no results. Finally the doctor came in and, along with a new nurse (who took over for the previous nurse a few minutes prior), helped us make some progress on the pushing, but determined that the head was too big for the cervix (the opening was too small) to make this work. That's

when the idea of the vacuum came up. We were all for it—beats a C-section for sure. We had no fears. We were aware that we'd end up with a temporary cone-head, but we just wanted the baby already. We didn't have an option between vacuum and forceps. We'd been told that the doctors will use whatever they are most comfortable with. When they started preparing the vacuum, they called in a few assistants from the NICU. That made us a little nervous because it indicated something could go wrong. After two pushes and five minutes later, our little coneheaded daughter came out. I don't remember much of anything. But once I saw the head, I turned to my wife and said, "Holy shit!" The bump on her head (I always called it a brioche because it was shaped like the little knob on the top of brioche bread) was gone within a few days.

—Jason, daughter 5 months

✳ ✳ ✳

Welcome to labor and delivery.

Most men think of themselves as experts when it comes to the vagina but know very little about labor and delivery. As the third trimester progresses, you'll hear a lot about the cervix, dilation, effacement,

The doctor wasn't there yet, just the nurse. The nurse told her to stop pushing, but my wife is like, "*I gotta get this thing out of there!*" I had one leg and her mom had the other leg. She was all out pushing at this point. The nurse commented that she had never seen a first-time birth go that quickly.
—Bob (son 17 months)

episiotomies, epidurals, natural birth, cesarean sections, crowning, pushing, episiotomies, and the placenta. I wasn't always sure what the doctors were talking about. Here's a quick summary of what's going to happen during labor and delivery and some insight into the terminology.

Imagine that the vagina is a road (call it Vagina Lane); a block or so up Vagina Lane is the cervix. The cervix is the opening to the uterus. Before pregnancy, the uterus is about the size of a pear. During pregnancy, the uterus grows to about a thousand times its original size. Think of a pregnant woman's uterus as a big balloon. The opening of the balloon is the cervix. For the past 38 weeks, the cervix has thickened, remained closed, and been sealed off with a mucous plug (as added protection).

The first stage of labor is when the cervix dilates (10 cm is fully dilated), thins out (this is called effacement), and opens up so the baby can move through it and into the birth canal (a.k.a. the vagina).

The second stage is when the baby enters the birth canal and is pushed into the world. If the baby is too big to pass through the birth canal, a doctor might perform an episiotomy (cutting the skin between the vagina and the anus). Once the baby is delivered, there's another stage.

The third and final stage of labor is the delivery of the placenta. The placenta is the organ that formed in the uterus through which the baby received nourishment from the mother. The umbilical cord is attached to the placenta.

STAGE 1: THE THREE PHASES

1. Early labor
2. Active labor
3. Transition

Early labor: The earliest signs of labor (a fitting name). Contractions become regular and uncomfortable (for her, not you); the cervix begins to dilate, assuming it hasn't already started. Contractions during early labor are generally five to ten minutes apart. Early labor can last days. Usually there is plenty of time to get to your caregiver. (I'm not a betting man, but I would bet $100 that everyone reading this will make it to the hospital or birthing center before giving birth. That's how rare it is to *not* make it to your destination.) Your health care provider will tell you when it's time to go to the hospital.

Active labor: This is when the real action starts. Contractions become more frequent and more intense (two to four minutes apart). The cervix goes from 3 cm to 7 cm during active labor. During active labor, the lessons from the birthing class start coming into play. You can begin to help with

> I was induced the first time, told I wasn't making progress (0 cm!) in the first four hours of horrendous contractions. The doctor told me I was going to have a C-section if I didn't progress in the next half hour. I told him to get the "F" out of my room and give himself an F-ing C-section.
>
> —*Amanda (expecting #5)*

> I was shocked when they told me to grab her leg. I thought, "Isn't there a nurse to do that?" Or at least someone who is getting paid to be there. After all, I'm paying ten grand to the hospital; I shouldn't have to hold anything.
>
> —*AJ (son 18 months)*

breathing, massaging her back, playing music, counting the timing of each contraction, suggesting birthing positions, helping her find a focal point, or staying far away (if she doesn't want you that close to her).

Transition: This is the fast and furious phase. The cervix will be completely dilated and effaced. Contractions can last a minute or longer. Some women get nauseous and might vomit during this phase. As the contractions increase with intensity, everyone will assume their positions. When my wife transitioned, the room did too. The bottom third of the bed was removed and the doctor and nurse assumed the position. It all moves very quickly. When she starts to transition, stay focused on being there for her. This is when you might encounter some serious verbal abuse—and no, don't answer her back. Just listen and take it like a man helping his partner through labor.

STAGE 2: THE BIRTH

It's time. The moment has arrived. Drum roll please…

The nurse told to me to grab a leg (my wife's, not the nurse's). My job was to hold her right leg (even though I'm a lefty) and help her through the contractions. Helping meant counting the contractions. I would tell her when each contraction was building, peaking, and ending. I followed the nurse's lead. We'd tell her, "Here comes another one, it's

> I felt like I had zero choice about cutting the umbilical cord. I initially declined, and said, "No, thanks," about three times, and then two nurses forced the skin scissors in my hand to cut.
>
> —*Todd (son 4 months)*

starting, get ready, push, okay, halfway through it, almost done, a little longer, okay, relax now... you're doing great..." Because she was hooked up to a monitor, I could see the contractions build, peak, and diminish on screen. Each contraction looked like a mountain on the monitor—building, building, peaking, and descending. She would rest between each contraction (about a minute or so). This part of the process is different for every couple. Every caregiver also has his or her own style of helping her through it.

During the birthing phase, the baby moves down the birth canal. Pushing can be long, tiring, and arduous. It can last for several minutes or several hours; labor typically lasts the longest with the first child (it's not nearly as long the second time).

As your pregnant partner pushes, the baby's head will start crowning. This is when the top of the head is visible through the vagina. Crowning is a surreal image. She'll push and then stop pushing and a little bit of the baby's head will be visible each time. This will be the first time you see the baby. Some guys don't want to look in that area. Personally, I was locked and in awe. I thought it was amazing. (I'll get to this more in Tip #87: Preg-Man-See, but seeing it was profound in the best way.) At one point, my daughter's head was completely out, but she was still one push away from being completely out. My wife looked down and said, "The baby looks like my brother." We didn't know if "it" was a boy or girl yet. I didn't see the family resemblance, but I didn't feel that was the time to discuss this with her. If your partner wants to look, make sure there's a mirror positioned so she can see the action (address this with the nurses and put it in your birth plan). For some women seeing the movement while pushing helps them concentrate.

During the birth you'll find out if the baby can fit through the birth canal. Sometimes the baby could be turned too far in one direction or be in the breech position (with the baby's buttocks or feet first). Sometimes the birth canal can be too narrow. The umbilical cord could be in a delicate position. Until she reaches the pushing part, you won't know. If you want to know what the pushing feels like, it's like bearing down to push out a bowel movement (but according to my wife, a hundred times harder). But whatever you do, *do not* push with your partner during the birth phase. (You'll give birth to something else.)

As you move through the birthing phase, your partner might need help with the final push. She's exhausted, hasn't eaten, and has been experiencing labor for hours; she might not be able to push any more. In some situations, forceps or a suction vacuum will be used to help with the final pushes. Your partner might need some help getting through the final stretch. If for any reason she can't push, don't make her feel bad about it. Do not pressure her. Do not force her. Do not make her feel guilty. It's exhausting—support her, encourage her, and listen to her.

As she is pushing, the doctor will work to make sure she doesn't have any vaginal tearing. If the baby can't make it through the birth canal without tearing, the doctor might opt to do an episiotomy. This means cutting the area between the anus and the vagina to make more room for the baby to pass through the birth canal. Discuss with your doctor beforehand if she does not want this, but usually it's done to prevent painful tearing. Once the baby and placenta are delivered, the doctor will stitch up any cuts or tears. Once the head is out, the rest of the baby comes fast. Then, the baby is born. This is when the umbilical cord is clamped, and you get to cut (or not cut). Sometimes the doctor will insist that you cut the cord. You can say "No" if you're not comfortable. After a quick hello, the baby is taken for some cleaning and testing, and mom begins stage 3.

STAGE 3: THE PLACENTA ARRIVES

Stage 3 threw me. No one ever talks about this phase. I had no idea there was a stage 3. While everyone is celebrating the birth of the baby, the placenta (the organ attached to the other end of the umbilical cord) is still inside your partner. On one end of the room, your partner is delivering the placenta. On the other side of the room, nurses are cleaning, testing, stamping feet, and doing the Apgar test (see Tip #89).

As the one who's supposed to be there for your partner, it can be a bit confusing where

> They hooked up an electronic fetal monitor to my wife and the baby. When my wife pushed, the baby's heart rate went nuts. I thought the baby was in terrible danger. Apparently, when I mentioned something to the nurse I was told that it's fairly normal.
>
> —*Eric (daughter 20 months)*

THE ELECTRONIC FETAL MONITOR:

During active labor, the baby's heart rate and your partner's contractions will be tracked through the use of an electronic fetal monitor. It works by placing two electronic disks (transducers) on her belly (elastic bands wrap around her torso to hold them in place). If experiencing a natural delivery (i.e., no pain medication), an electronic fetal monitor may not be used because it restricts movement. If having an epidural, a monitor will be in use throughout the labor.

you should go—do you videotape the baby? Snap photos? Or do you stick with the mom and help her get over the final stage? I stuck with the baby and kept an eye on my wife. I felt like this was the right thing to do at the time, but never having talked about it, a part of me felt like I was abandoning her. I explained this to her after the delivery, but it would have been nice to have talked about this part of the process beforehand. She didn't have a problem with it, but I know other women have. Consider making a plan so that she doesn't feel like you're running off with the baby.

Once the placenta is delivered, the doctor will clean up your partner and make sure everything is as it should be. If you have a second, check out the placenta. It was the home base for baby; it's what's nourished him or her. Some people will take the placenta home and plant it in the backyard. Other people will cook it. We didn't eat it, cook it, or smoke it and turn it into placenta jerky, but I did take a picture of it. And you can see that picture at www.DadsPregnant.com. (Thank you to my wife for allowing me to post the picture of the placenta.)

THE BOTTOM LINE:
Stage 4. The Celebration

Tip #85
THE C-SECTION SECTION: About One-Third of New Dads Will See It This Way

THE TIP:
It was seven minutes from the time I sat down until she was born. Had I known it would go so fast, I wouldn't have waited to pee.

THE STORY:
We weren't planning on a C-section delivery. The doctor explained to me that the labor stalled at 4 cm dilation. We prepped and signed the forms. By 7:30 a.m. the paperwork was done. I asked if I would be allowed in the operating room. I was told "Yes." I was then given a plastic kit with scrubs (pants, a mask, and hat). They didn't give me any instructions other than, "We'll get you when we're ready." My wife was wheeled for prep and I changed into my scrubs. All alone, I was left sitting

in the labor and delivery room by myself. I had to pee, so I went into the bathroom for a second. From 9:30 a.m. to 9:39 a.m., I sat in the room waiting—I imagined that they came to get me while I was in the bathroom, and I missed the delivery. Finally, they came for me at 9:40 a.m. By 9:42 a.m., I was standing in a brightly lit operating room looking at my wife who was splayed out as if she was being crucified. A drape was set up a few inches below her chin so she couldn't see what was happening. I sat down in the chair next to her—also behind the drape. There was a resident to my right, the doctor on the other side, and four nurses and the anesthesiologist in the room. They told me it was going to go fast and that really soon I'm going to be a dad. That's when I started to get nervous. It was hard to breathe with the mask. I kept thinking of all the stories of guys passing out and it made me think about passing out. My heart started racing. The doctor told me, "Any minute now." I then heard them say, "Oh look at the chubby cheeks." They told me to stand up and said, "You have a beautiful girl." All I remember is locking in on her face and seeing them pulling her out. I was locked on her eyes. After the delivery, they took her across the room, wiped her down, weighed her, and made sure she was doing well. About five minutes later, they called me over to meet her and cut a few inches off of the umbilical cord. She was on the scale weighing in at 8 pounds, 4 ounces. The nurses then wrapped her up and I carried her over to my wife. The whole time my wife hadn't seen her. I got to see her first. That was special. I walked over to my wife and handed her our daughter. It was seven minutes from the time I sat down until she was born.

—Anthony, daughter 2 weeks

✳ ✳ ✳

I was delivered via C-section before it was trendy to have a C-section. I like to think of my mom as a trendsetter.

Seriously, according to the Centers for Disease Control, 29.1 percent of all U.S. births in in 2004 were delivered via C-section. Whether she's planning for a vaginal or C-section delivery ask the doctor to walk you through the procedure. Ask if you'll be in the room the whole time. Ask if she will get to hold the baby right away. Ask whatever questions are on your mind. If it's an unplanned C-section, make sure to support your partner. Be flexible and adjust your plan. Labor is unpredictable— your support of your partner needs to be unwavering.

You might be planning to have a C-section delivery. You might be planning for a vaginal birth. The reasons for the C-sections vary—some are because of medical issues, some due to the position of

First child was an emergency C-section. Second was a planned C-section. She liked the second one better. It was cool to see her insides put on top of her stomach. Dad always wanted me to follow in his footsteps and be a doctor.
—Jeff (daughter 10 months, son 5½ years)

The most surprising part of labor was how fast it went. She had a scheduled C-section. It was over in ten minutes.
—Todd (son 4 months)

the baby, some due to developing situations, and some for convenience. (This way no one misses the game on TV.) Whether or not you're planning a C-section, here are some things to keep in mind:

1. An epidural or spinal block is the most common form of medication. Your partner will most likely be awake and alert during the procedure. They will also insert a catheter into her urethra (to drain urine). See Tip #79 for more on pain meds.

2. Most facilities will allow you in the operating room during the procedure. You'll scrub in and wear the appropriate clothes. If it's an emergency C-section or if your partner is under a general anesthesia (meaning she's not awake), you might not be allowed inside.

3. Once in the operating room, they will most likely position a screen to keep you from watching the early part of the procedure. If you want to see the action, ask to have the screen lowered when the baby leaves the womb. You might be allowed to stand and see the procedure.

4. Recovery is longer than with a vaginal birth. It can be a three- or four-day hospital stay. This is major surgery, and with any major surgery there is an increased risk of infection and other complications. Things like walking up stairs and picking up the baby should be avoided afterward.

The amount of blood that gushed out after the initial C-section incision freaked me out. It looked like so much, like we were in trouble. I later found out it wasn't all that much.

—*Anonymous*

5. A C-section isn't a reflection on a mom doing something right or wrong. If it's something that needs to happen, allow it to happen. Sometimes the cervix won't thin or dilate, or the baby is too big, or too excited, or in distress. Sometimes mom can be in distress.

THE BOTTOM LINE:
Ask your doctor to walk you through the procedure, even if it's not part of the birth plan. If there is an emergency, there won't be time to discuss it.

Tip #86
THE CONEHEAD: And Other Newborn Oddities

THE TIP:
Imagine your baby's head getting squeezed out of a tiny hole. Then watch the *Coneheads* movie. That's what you should expect.

THE STORY:
I've got one of my wife's legs on my shoulder and the nurse had her other leg on her shoulder. My wife kept looking at me because the expression on my face was like, "What's going on here?" I tried to keep a straight face. After my son fully came out, I told her he had such a conehead that the money we put aside for college was

going to have to go toward plastic surgery. He looked like he came straight out of the movie. Thank God a day or two later, the conehead went down. With a hat on his head, he looked like a cute baby. Without the hat, his head was scary looking. My daughter was smaller, and I don't think she was affected by going through the birth canal. But my son had such a big head that squeezing out made it look longer and pretty ugly. We had no expectations about how the baby would look, and the conehead shocked me.

—Corey, son 2½ years, daughter 8 months

✳ ✳ ✳

Getting pushed through the cervix and being forced down the birth canal is like getting pushed through a crowded bar on New Year's Eve. Newborn babies are squeezed, pushed, pulled, suctioned, cut (from the cord), forcepped, and forced from a liquid world to dry land. Their lungs literally go from breathing fluid one second to breathing air the next. Their skin can be coated with a white pasty substance. They might have splotches on their skin from the ride down Vagina Lane. They might have hair in strange places. Their faces can appear swollen. Their heads are elongated.

While childbirth is absolutely beautiful, a newborn out of the womb has a look of her own—like a boxer who just went fifteen rounds. You will think the baby is beautiful, but the conehead or some other newborn vanity issue might freak you out. If the medical staff isn't worried, then don't be worried. I still have a hard time understanding how this could be normal, but coneheads are normal.

My daughter had the most elongated head I've ever seen. One time my wife pushed and stopped while my daughter's head was halfway through the opening. The entire top of her head was pushing out like an eraser on top of a pencil. I wanted to push her head out, but pushing would have left me with other problems. After a couple more contractions and pushes, my daughter's head cleared. By this time, her head was completely elongated. I asked the doctor if this was normal. I couldn't imagine how this could be normal. The doctor explained that the baby's skull plates are soft and able to shift during delivery. The bones have yet to harden or fuse. This flexibility allows the skull to pass through the birth canal. After a few hours of relaxation, my daughter's head was looking rounder. The next day, she no longer had that conehead.

An elongated head was just one of several things no one warned me about. When your kid makes his or her first appearance, you might be surprised that the baby doesn't look like you expected. Some things to prepare for include the following:

- The baby's skin could be covered with grayish greasy paste. This is called vernix, and it protects the baby's skin in the fluid environment. There might also be some newborn acne, red splotches, and wear and tear from birth.

- The baby's head might be misshapen and bruised. The skull plates shift during birth, allowing the head to travel safely down the birth canal. Don't worry about this hurting the brain—again, a conehead is normal.
- Your baby's eyes will look puffy. There might be broken blood vessels on the eyelids from the pushing. Eyes might have a hard time opening. Focusing on objects more than a few inches away could make the baby appear cross-eyed.
- If you have a boy, his genitals will look huge. (Yes, I know you're proud, but it's temporary.) If you have a girl, there will be swelling in the genital area too. The increase in hormones causes this to happen, and it's normal.
- The belly button has the remains of the umbilical cord hanging out (it's clipped). The cord will eventually fall off naturally (or the doctor will remove it), but it may look a little strange, especially with the clamp attached to it.
- The baby's skin color might look a little blue, yellow, red, or another shade of the rainbow. If the shade varies from your shade, ask your doctor about it. High levels of bilirubin will give the skin a jaundiced (yellow) look; if it's really low they might put your baby under a blue light.

THE BOTTOM LINE:

Even the most coneheaded, puffy-eyed, greasy-feeling, huge-scrotumed, hairy baby is beautiful.

Tip #87

THE TIP:

Get in there as much as you can, enjoy it, and expect to be surprised.

THE STORY:

During labor, I saw something my wife tried to prepare me for, but still, I wasn't prepared. I was standing over the doctor's shoulder during the heavy pushing. I wanted to see it all. She had been pushing for a good twenty minutes and I could start to see the head come out. In the middle of one of the intense contractions I saw a couple of pieces of poop drop out. The doctor waited until my wife finished the contraction and casually moved it to the side. To them, it was just part of doing business and no big concern. My wife told me this might happen, but it still surprised me. It didn't bother me though. With the level of excitement involved with the birth, it paled in comparison when all was said and done. Being there and watching the baby coming out was the most exciting moment of my entire life. I had the best seat in the house—I would definitely recommend it. The crowning moment was when my daughter came into the world. I couldn't imagine not seeing the whole thing.

—Scot, daughter 14 months

✳ ✳ ✳

To look or not to look? That's the question.

It's hard for a guy to not look at a naked woman, but this isn't a naked woman. This is a naked woman with a baby coming out of her vagina. That might freak you out—and yes, that's a natural reaction. Considering we are the first generation of dads in the delivery room, we're the ones who are seeing it for the first time. What you decide is a personal decision, but I can tell you that what you imagine you will see and what you will actually see (should you look) are entirely different.

I didn't know if I was going to look, but I ended up looking. In fact, I couldn't take my eyes away from it. It was surreal. Looking didn't ruin it for me. I wasn't scared of her vagina or intimidated following the birth. If anything, I was even more intrigued. This once sexual part of her body was truly transformed into something entirely different. And that wasn't a bad thing because it changed back following the

Hell yes, I looked. It was amazing. The most intense and emotional experience of my life by far.

—Eric (daughter 22 months)

It's an overall surreal and remarkable experience but you do not need to have the aftermath burned in your brain.

—Mike (son 12 months)

birth. I mentioned this in Tip #9, the "GUYne" tip, but there is a distinct difference between the vagina you fell in love with and the vagina that gives birth to your child. The SV (sex vagina) is what you know and love. The BV (birthing vagina) is what you'll see if you look.

What I saw and felt while watching my daughter being born into this world was the most powerful moment of my life. I wouldn't have wanted to look anywhere else. I've talked to guys who didn't want that image burned into their minds and guys who are thrilled the image is forever burned into their minds. For me:

- Looking was *not* disgusting.
- Looking was *not* a turnoff.
- Looking was *not* damaging.

Going into labor, my wife was 100 percent sure she didn't want me to look. I didn't argue. By the time we hit transition, she was *not* focused on where I was looking. And she was looking. As labor progressed, she even used a mirror (another thing she didn't think she'd want) so she could see the pushing. The mirror was motivating because she could see her pushing progress (something I've also heard from other women). It's like having a rearview mirror, but you're not looking at the rear view. Even the way she saw her vagina

Yes and I am happy that I watched it all. Why wouldn't I want to? It was a once-in-a-lifetime chance to see this, which also happens to be kind of a miracle!

—*Dan (son 4 months)*

changed. What she thought she was going to want and what she wanted at the time of delivery were two different things.

Until you're there, you don't know. Some guys won't look and will never look—but I have to tell you that it's just about the most amazing thing I've ever seen in my life. It didn't look anything like I imagined. I didn't pass out. I didn't scream. And it was not a turnoff. In fact, we're in the second trimester of baby #2, so clearly we were able to reconnect.

THE BOTTOM LINE:
You've never seen anything like it in your life—I guarantee it.

Tip #88
LIGHTS, CAMERA, ACTION!: A Once-in-a-Lifetime Shot at the Perfect Shot

THE TIP:
Don't worry about cutting the cord—worry about getting the shot.

THE STORY:
There was this great shot of my son on the scale where his wiener wasn't visible. I needed to get the same shot of our second baby. When the baby came out, the doctor kept asking me if I wanted to cut the cord. I told him I didn't want to cut it. I felt a lot of pressure to get

the video, and there are missed shots that you can never get back. He asked me again. I said, "I'm trying to get a shot here. I can't cut the cord. I don't want to cut the cord. I'll be spending my life with the baby and cutting the cord isn't as important as getting this shot." All I wanted was to get the shot. I got the shot. I also made sure to be careful what I shot. Last time I accidentally took a picture of something I didn't realize. We load all our pictures into the computer's screensaver, which rotates through about a thousand shots. One day we had some friends over, and I ran into the other room to get something when I saw a picture of my wife completely naked in the delivery room. I looked to see if anyone else saw it and I was safe. I deleted it so that no one ever knew. It could have been a disaster.

—*Gary, sons 8 months and 3½ years*

＊ ＊ ＊

The big question: Does an adult man or woman really need to see a video of him- or herself being pulled out of his mother's vagina? That's a question only an adult who has seen videos of his or her birth can answer. As of right now, there are no adults who can answer that question because videotaping

Forget the video camera. We brought one, thinking we'd videotape the birth from some prime angle where my wife would look beautiful and you wouldn't see her persqueeter. But no such angle exists in reality.

—*Eric (son 18 months)*

birth is a fairly recent trend. Traumatic or dramatic—I'm not sure.

Never before have there been more opportunities to capture the images of the first minutes of your baby's life. As someone who spends a lot of time videotaping family moments, I know that there's a dramatic difference between seeing something with my own eyes and seeing something through the lens of the camera. I'm so grateful that the hospital had a policy that prohibited videotaping the actual birth. The rules allowed us to take photos and videos before and immediately following the birth, but not during it. Even if there wasn't a policy prohibiting it, I can't imagine that I'd want to do it after I thought it through. Here are five reasons why:

1. Operating a video camera means having to concentrate on something other than her. She deserves all the attention.
2. Even if I set the camera up on a tripod on a static shot, I would have to worry about the tape, battery, graphic shots, or knocking it over.
3. Videotaping before and after the moment can capture the essence of the moment.
4. I have enough video to show at special events.
5. Some things are better left to the imagination.

My job for the second was to hold the camera, the camcorder, and her leg and to make sure the mirror was angled right for her.

—Jim (daughter 2 months, son 3¼ years)

If you do decide to take pictures or video, make sure you have a plan. Ask your partner what she's comfortable with. If she resists, explain that you can put this together in a scrapbook page for the baby. It's not for you, it's for him or her. When it comes to the actual birth, make sure she knows that you might have to leave her side. If you want to capture pictures of the baby being weighed, stamped, and washed, you're going to have to go to the other side of the room while she's in the midst of stage 3. The most important thing is that documenting the birth doesn't take away from her level of comfort and relaxation. Talking about it and having a plan will help avoid any accidental asshole moments on your part.

THE EQUIPMENT

If there has ever been a time to warrant shopping for elec-

THE RIGHT EQUIPMENT:

Consider getting a WiFi digital camera. These cameras allow you to download photos without memory cards or USB cables. You point, shoot, and then send your pictures to your computer or a photo website.

Get a bigger memory card and avoid having to be selective about the photos you want to take. Just point and shoot again and again.

If purchasing a new video camera, consider getting one that records

tronics, this is it. Make her a deal—you'll go to Best Buy and she'll go to Babies 'R' Us, and you'll meet back in two hours. She can pick you up. If you don't have a digital camera, consider getting one along with onto an internal hard drive that can be downloaded to your computer. Avoid having to purchase and keep track of digital videotapes. Purchase two hard drives (one to download videos to and one to back up the videos).

a memory card with huge capacity (which is inexpensive). You want the flexibility to take as many pictures as you want. With digital technology, even the worst photographer has the opportunity to take hundreds of crappy photos in search of one good one. The chances of getting that one good one are high when you take a thousand shots within a ten-minute window.

If you don't want to worry about downloading pictures or dealing with a memory card, consider getting a WiFi camera. A new generation of cameras allows you to snap photos and then download them to a computer, a cellular network, or the Internet without having to remove a memory card or bring a USB cable. Once you snap the photo, you can send it within minutes.

If you don't own a video camera or want a new video camera, this is a great time to do it. The prices are inexpensive compared to even a year ago. For this next pregnancy, I'm contemplating a camera with an internal hard drive. This way, I won't have to worry about keeping track of digital videotapes and downloading them. If you have a video camera with a hard drive, you can download videos directly to your computer and to a backup hard drive. The general rule is that for every gigabyte, you get one hour of video (this can vary). As for downloading, memory prices have also decreased dramatically. You can find a 160-gigabyte hard drive for less than $100 (probably less by the time this book prints). When it comes to finding the best camera and best deal, shop around and then consider buying online (you can avoid the sales tax). Just make sure to buy from a reputable retailer that guarantees its products. Make sure your computer is compatible with your new equipment.

PLAN YOUR SHOOT:

Investigate the facility's policies when it comes to video and photos.

Discuss what will happen once the baby is born. (Will you stay by her side or snap photos of the baby?)

Ask your doctor or midwife if he or she has any requests. Make sure whatever you're doing isn't going to get in the way.

One more thing worth mentioning: It's also a good idea to bring your laptop with you to the hospital (if you have one). When things settle down, you can download the pictures and send them to your list of contacts. In just a few hours following the birth you can send an email birth announcement, post the photo on your Facebook profile, or send a photo via your phone.

THE BOTTOM LINE:
If you do videotape the entire birth from all angles with tight close-ups in high definition, this could be a fantastic video to show your son's or daughter's future significant others to promote birth control.

Tip #89
WHAT HAPPENS NEXT?: Newborn Care, Crowd Control, and Sleep

THE TIP:
When the baby is born, skin-to-skin contact is the best way to bond.

THE STORY:
It was by chance that I came across kangaroo care when I was doing research on a project. Kangaroo care is based on how kangaroos use skin-to-skin contact to comfort newborns. It can be chest-to-chest or

any skin-to-skin contact, and it helps regulate the baby's temperature and heart rate. It's soothing. As soon as he was in the room I would open my shirt and lay him on my chest. It was an amazing experience and connection. He seemed to be comforted by me—it was profound that he could be comforted by me. There were so many benefits to it. When we were in the hospital, the nurses would come into the room and notice me and say, "Oh, kangaroo care!" I can't recommend it enough.

—Todd, son 3 months

＊＊＊

Once the baby is born, things will happen.

ONCE THE BABY IS BORN

If she has a vaginal delivery, your newborn will be taken over to another area of the room and examined after the birth. You can decide whether or not you want to cut the cord. Before the baby is examined following the birth, the mom can request to hold the baby. If you are following the Bradley Method

The family is going to be needy—people may come over too much. The hospital room is very small, and people just stand around watching you and the baby.

—Gary (sons 8 months and 3½ years)

He didn't spend the night with me either time. The room was too small, it wasn't private, and I just wanted to sleep.

—Collette
(daughters 5 months and 5 years)

or the Lamaze philosophy, immediate contact with the mother following delivery is encouraged. This means the moment the baby is born, skin-to-skin contact and comfort is the chosen approach. If nursing, breastfeeding as soon as possible is another component of aftercare. Whatever you and your partner want to have happen, make sure you communicate this to your doctor, midwife, and medical team. If having a C-section, ask the doctor to walk you through the aftercare before the procedure. It can vary based on the hospital.

After the birth, the doctor showed our daughter to my wife and then the nurses took the baby to another area of the room where they examined her, performed the Apgar test, cleaned her off, put a bracelet on her ankle, and stamped her feet. Since we never discussed the aftercare, we just went with the flow. But if you have preferences, you can change the flow. It's your delivery and your child.

The following are standard tests and procedures that will be conducted once your newborn arrives (Source: www.4women.gov). Ask your caregiver to go over the specifics; procedures can vary based on local laws and hospital procedures. If you are uncomfortable with any part of a procedure, discuss it with your caregiver.

I slept on the uncomfortable pullout. On the last night they kicked our daughter out of the nursery and into our room because she was crying. We got no sleep. After the nurse kicked our daughter out of the nursery we walked by the window and saw the empty nursery and her playing solitaire on the computer.

—*David (daughter 6 months)*

Apgar Evaluation: The Apgar test is a quick way for doctors to figure out if the baby is healthy or needs extra medical care. Apgar tests are usually done twice: one minute after birth and again five minutes after birth. Doctors and nurses measure five signs of the baby's condition:

- Heart rate
- Breathing
- Activity and muscle tone
- Reflexes
- Skin color

Apgar scores range from 0 to 10. A baby who scores 7 or more is considered very healthy. But a lower score doesn't always mean there is something wrong. Perfectly healthy babies often have low Apgar scores in the first minute of life. In more than 98 percent of cases, the Apgar score reaches 7 after five minutes of life. When it does not, the baby needs medical care and close monitoring.

Eye Care: The Centers for Disease Control and Prevention (CDC) recommend that all newborns receive eye drops or ointment to prevent infections they can acquire during delivery. Sexually transmitted diseases (STDs) including gonorrhea and chlamydia are a main cause of newborn eye infections. These infections can cause blindness when left untreated.

Silver nitrate, erythromycin, and tetracycline are the three medicines used in newborns' eyes (erythromycin is mostly used these days). These medicines can sting and/or blur the baby's vision, so you may want to talk to your caregiver for more details. Some parents question whether this treatment is really necessary. Many women at low risk for STDs do not want their newborns to receive eye medicine, but there is no evidence to suggest that this medicine harms the baby. It is important to note that even pregnant women who test negative for STDs may get an infection by the time of delivery. Plus, most women with gonorrhea and/or chlamydia don't know it because they have no symptoms. The antibiotic eye ointments may also help prevent infection with other bacteria, besides the ones that cause STDs.

Vitamin K Shot: The American Academy of Pediatrics recommends that all newborns receive a shot of vitamin K in the upper leg. Newborns usually have low levels of vitamin K in their bodies. This vitamin is necessary for blood clotting. Low levels of vitamin K can cause a rare but serious bleeding problem. Research shows that vitamin K shots prevent dangerous bleeding in newborns. Newborns probably feel pain when the shot is given, but babies don't seem to have any discomfort afterwards.

Newborn Metabolic Screening: Doctors or nurses prick your baby's heel to take a tiny sample of blood. They use this blood to test for many diseases. All fifty states require testing for at least two disorders: phenylketonuria and congenital hypothyroidism. But many states test for up to thirty different diseases. All of these problems are impossible to spot without a blood test. And if left untreated they can cause mental retardation and even death. The March of Dimes recommends that all newborns be tested for at least twenty-nine diseases, even if your state doesn't require it.

Hearing Screening: Many hospitals perform newborn hearing screenings. Tiny earphones or microphones are used to monitor how the baby reacts to sounds. Newborn hearing tests can detect hearing problems early, which can help cut the risk of serious language and speech problems. Universal hearing screening is recommended by the AAP. These tests measure brainwaves though and don't measure a baby's reaction to sound in the traditional sense.

Hepatitis B Vaccine: Most hospitals now suggest that newborns get a vaccine to protect against the hepatitis B virus (HBV). The hepatitis B vaccine is a series of three different shots. The second and last shot should be given before 18 months of age.

MANAGING MOM'S AND BABY'S AFTERCARE

Once the baby is born, you are in charge of making sure your partner and the baby are getting the care they need. (I know you're tired and need to relax, but there's just a little more you need to do.) If you do not want the baby to undergo a particular test or procedure, tell the medical team before the birth; then, just in case, stick with the baby once it's born. The only way to assure that the care you desire is administered is to be there while care is being administered. The only exception would be if there's an emergency. When it comes to your partner's recovery, don't be so quick to leave her and go home. See Tip #80 about being her advocate. The first 24 to 48 hours are important for you to be there to make sure she's comfortable. While chances are small that there will be complications following delivery, it's worth sticking around.

MANAGING THE CROWDS

Once the baby is born, people will want to come by. Your partner will be excited and exhausted—it's been a long day. Again, you are the guy working the door. The room is small, and she's going to need to rest. Also, you're going to want time to get to know how the baby works and bond as a family. (Kangaroo care is great.) Doing things like changing diapers, feeding the baby, caring for the umbilical stump, burping the baby, and soothing the baby are things the nurses can help you with.

Once the baby is born, send out an email (using a list you've prepared) and share the specifics. You can briefly mention everything about the baby, "Mom is doing great—very tired, but great. I'll be in touch with more updates in the next few days." If everyone knows all is well and that she's tired, that should help to keep the calls to a minimum. When people call asking to visit, it might be a good idea to have them come by after she gets home, given that you're only in the hospital for two days and visiting hours are limited. If people want to do something nice, suggest that they bring over lunch or dinner (if you're comfortable asking). If she wants visitors, make sure to let the visitors know that she's tired but would *never* tell them. One more thing, when you do have visitors, ask them

After the baby is born, they will:
- Measure the newborn's weight, length, and head.
- Take the baby's temperature.
- Measure his breathing and heart rate.
- Give the baby a bath and clean the umbilical cord stump.

If you're worried about the baby being away from you because of security reasons, ask the hospital what procedures are in place. Our hospital had a bracelet system that activated an alarm if the baby was taken out of the maternity ward.

to wash their hands when they come in, especially if they want to hold the baby. The nurses wash up, so should everyone else.

WHERE BABY SLEEPS AT NIGHT

Where your newborn sleeps in the hospital will be one issue. Most likely, you will either have the option of having the baby sleep in the room with mom (known as "rooming in") or having the baby sleep in the nursery. If the baby is nursing (breast-feeding) and sleeping in the nursery, a nurse will bring the baby to mom when the baby gets hungry. If the baby is bottle-fed, the mom doesn't have to do the feeding. You might want to have the baby in the room to spend the night together as a family, which makes sense. However you will share many nights as a family at home, but you also won't have a lot of good nights' sleep or a night nurse to take care of your baby. A night nurse is a luxury. We quickly realized that the nursery was a *great* thing. Whatever your philosophy, know that you have an option. We learned that we could be loving parents and still have our daughter sleep in the nursery.

WHERE YOU SLEEP AT NIGHT

Given that fathers have historically not been an intricate part of the birthing process, many hospitals were not built to accommodate fathers spending the night with their partners following birth. If sharing a room with another patient, the father might not have the option of spending the night. Should the rules allow you to spend the night in the room, you may have to sleep on a chair, a couch, or a cot. Investigate this beforehand when selecting a birthing facility. If you do spend the night and are uncomfortable, don't tell her about it. I made the mistake of complaining. After giving birth, she doesn't want to hear you complain.

THE BOTTOM LINE:

Let the nurses help as much as possible. Don't be a hero. Once you go home, you'll miss them (unless you take one home).

Tip #90
LEAVING THE HOSPITAL: Taking Everything You Can Fit through the Door

THE TIP:
Stockpile as you go and check the supply closet door. You might just find yourself in the middle of Fort Knox.

THE STORY:
We raided the place. I even snuck into the supply room. Everyone told us we should clean out the supply cart because it will be replenished. I cleaned it out and stockpiled stuff in bags then took it home nightly. Every morning they would refill the cart and I would stockpile again. One time when I went to get ice, I noticed the supply room door near the kitchen. It's always under tight lock and key. I checked the door and somehow it opened. I was like "Ooooohhhhhhhhh, all this stuff." It was like raiding Fort Knox. I went to town grabbing wipes, diapers, swaddle blankets, onesies, changing pads, formula—as much formula as I could take with me. The next day I tried the door again; they had closed it, but not before I had gotten what must have been two weeks' worth of supplies.

Take extra bags and slowly fill your car with all their goodies! The nurses told me to! Take some snacks!
—*Nancy (daughter 15 months)*

—*David, daughter 6 months*

✷ ✷ ✷

This is why you packed an extra bag—to take things. When you leave the hospital you're going to want to take everything home that fits through the door. Check with the nurses to see what you can take in terms of supplies. (Do not take the nurses, that's called kidnapping.) Some supplies are meant to be taken (others are not and your insurance provider might bill you). Even if you have to pay for something you take, your insurance company might end up covering the bill as a special gift to you (also called a mistake).

Do not be shy about hoarding supplies. They expect it. Hospitals have lots of things that are hard to find in the outside world. Even if you can get these things outside, it's better to have as much of it as possible when you get home. Newborn shirts that snap on the side (to avoid rubbing the umbilical stump), receiving blankets for swaddling, diapers, diaper cream, blankets, maxi pads, alcohol pads, changing pads, gauze pads, icepacks, bottles (the 2-ounce ones are hard to find), blankets, formula (for now or later), and whatever else catches your eye—these are all things you should take with you. I'm not saying to steal anything, just take it—and if they stop you, just say, "Oh, sorry."

One additional bit of advice for when you're hoarding and stockpiling—ask for more (and they actually did give us more). By the time we were ready to leave, we had

We finally get home for the first time with our son and I realized I left the connection to the breast pump at the hospital and she needed to pump. I had to get back in my car and turn around and drive back by myself.

—Irl (son 22 months, expecting 28 weeks)

three bags' worth of supplies. We asked the nurses for more. And five minutes later, the nurse walked in with more. Ask and you shall receive—stuff or dirty looks.

Do not leave anything behind! Just make sure you go through the list of what you brought and check it off as you pack up to leave. Should you leave something behind, there's a good chance you'll have to go back to get it. And the last thing you're going to want to do is drive back to the hospital after driving home. This will be especially true if you've raided the place and still somehow managed to leave something behind.

One more reminder: Remember that in order to get out the door and in the getaway car with your stuff you'll need an infant car seat—it's required by law. If you haven't installed the car seat by week 35, do it. Usually the hospital can't help you with the installation. Make sure to follow the instructions and get it checked at a child seat fitting station. You don't want to be figuring out how to install the seat while your wife and newborn are waiting in the lobby for you to pull up in the getaway car (see Tip #64 for information on the car seat and a link to find child seat fitting locations).

THE BOTTOM LINE:

Take everything you can. If you need to leave this book behind because you don't have room for it, I understand. Get another one later.

Tip #91

THE TIP:
It just might be one of the most paranoid, surreal, mind-altering rides of your life. It will leave you on the edge of the driver's seat.

THE STORY:
The drive home was surreal, and I was paranoid. I was looking at all the other drivers acting as if they should know that I'm driving my child home for the first time. I'm like, "Don't you know I have a kid in the car?!" I thought braking hard would break the kid. I avoided hitting any bumps. I was driving with extreme caution. My wife and I were giddy, just cracking up. We were like "We're driving and there's a kid in our backseat." We had no idea what we were doing. To this day I drive differently when he's in the car. I drive slower, more cautiously, and much more deliberately, but I'm never as paranoid or hypersensitive as that day we put our son in the car for the very first time and took him home from the hospital. It was a drive more intense than drivers ed. I was on the edge of my seat and on the edge of my senses.

—Bob, son 17 months

* * *

It might happen to you on the ride to the hospital, but most likely, it will happen on the ride home from the hospital with your new family.

You'll signal with precision, follow at a safe distance, stop at yellow lights as if they are red, yield, give the right of way, allow cars to merge in front of you, and let people cut you off without speeding up to give them a dirty look. Lane changes will be executed with extreme precision. Stop signs will mean coming to a complete stop. Acceleration and braking will be as smooth as butter. You will follow the posted speed limit minus 5 miles per hour. Anyone passing, driving too fast, or looking at you the wrong way will stir your anger—the nerve of someone to jeopardize your family's safety when all you're trying to do is drive! You've never had more precious cargo.

The drive home will be like none other. What this drive really means is:

- You are in control.
- You are at the wheel.
- You are responsible…for this child's safety, security, and well-being.

The moment you take the wheel and drive away is the moment you realize how dangerous the world can be, how much you want to protect your child from it, and how little control you have over it. The drive home isn't about operating a vehicle. It's about feeling what it means to be a father behind the wheel for the first time.

P.S. Sorry if I was ever "the other guy" driving like an asshole. I had no idea you were coming home from the hospital.

THE BOTTOM LINE:
Welcome to life behind the wheel as a new dad. It's great to have you here…

13

AFTER THE BABY IS BORN

The Fourth Trimester Begins

Tip #92
WHAT NO ONE TELLS NEW DADS: The Most Honest
Advice You're Going to Get

THE TIP:
It might not be a magical mystical experience right
away. Don't feel bad for not feeling that right away. It
will be spectacular in a few months.

THE STORY:
The coolest moment was the delivery. But the first
two months were extremely stressful and exhausting
for me. I didn't know that it's normal not to feel that

magical sense. The whole time, everyone kept telling me how great it is. Right after my son was born, it was a huge adjustment—I was in shock-and-survival mode. I was just doing whatever I could for the first two or three months. I felt an overwhelming sense of responsibility. People at work were telling me to cherish the time. I wanted to slap those people after getting two hours of sleep and feeling completely exhausted. I snapped at a few people telling them it's really not that great. But it does get better. I can't emphasize that enough—it can take a few months until you're more confident and comfortable and in a routine. It all gets better, and it speeds up. I know that it's the last thing you want to hear for the first two or three months. I was bitter about it. Allow yourself to feel whatever you need to feel and know it will pass, and it will be better—it will be spectacular. For me, it took time. It had nothing to do with loving my kid; it was about a monumental transition, a new lifestyle, and an unprecedented sense of responsibility.

—*Josh, son 18 months*

* * *

> What was interesting and took a while for me to understand was that my wife immediately had a love for and attachment to our new baby; whereas it took me a lot longer to truly love the baby in that way.
>
> —*Don (son 8 months)*

When it comes to the expectant father experience, we don't have much of an oral history. We've only been allowed inside the delivery room for a little over thirty years. We are the first generation on the front line. What we're seeing, feeling, and experiencing is completely new—it's big. Each one of us is an orator who will help our friends, family, and future generations understand what's coming their way. Given what a new father goes through during the pregnancy, and then in labor and delivery, it makes sense that we can't articulate what we've been through other than telling our fellow man, "Things will change."

When guys give other guys advice about being a new dad, it's mainly about how things are going to change. (That's been a constant theme running throughout this book.) But their advice is rarely about how things will change for the better. It's more of an ominous warning as if a storm is heading your way and there's nothing you can do but stand there helplessly as the winds of change reach hurricane proportions.

I couldn't disagree more.

I don't disagree that things will change, but I do disagree that there is nothing we can do to prepare for this impending change. One reason the change is so dramatic and so hard to prepare for is that we're not told specifically what will change and how to prepare for the specific changes. If we knew what would change, we could prepare for it before it happens. Like a storm rolling in, we could board up the houses, put down sandbags to

> Your life as you know it is done. What I didn't count on, however, is how gladly and how easily I let my old life go, without a second thought. The kid makes it all worthwhile.
>
> —*Eric (son 9 months)*

prevent flooding, reinforce the levies, load up on supplies, and hopefully minimize the damage.

What if:

- We were told what will change when we have a baby?
- We could actively prepare for the change before it happens?
- We supported one another during change and shared what worked for us and what we learned along the way?

The answer is that it would be much easier to manage such a huge change. We could have much more fun managing the change. We could learn from one another and figure this out so that it doesn't have to be so daunting and ominous. Ultimately, we could anticipate, prepare, and weather the storm of change without getting knocked off our feet. Half the time, just knowing what is coming makes it easier to face.

As a second-time father, I can tell you that this time around I'm not as anxious. I know what is coming; I know what changes to expect. But I also know the first time around I didn't do anything to prepare in advance. I just stood there in the middle of the field, clueless, and exposed to the elements. Had I known what was coming my way I could have been ready.

Get at least one book. Stay ahead of the timeline. Find a guru, someone who has been there before and who can answer questions, give definitions, and share recommendations.

—Dan (son 4 months)

As you enter the next stage of this experience, things will

change. I've listed some of the things that will change and how to prepare for these changes. These are just a few suggestions. The idea is that if you know these things are coming, you can do whatever fits your personality to anticipate, face, embrace, and appreciate these changes as this experience reveals itself to you in real time.

CHANGES YOU CAN EXPECT

THE CHANGE: You'll get less attention from her.
THE ACTION PLAN: Plan how you'll be involved. Talk to her about what your roles will be. Ask her what she wants your role to be. Take a parenting class together. Pick up the book *The Happiest Baby on the Block* by Dr. Harvey Karp (more in Tip #93). Do something to be involved. Instead of watching the game or doing something on your own, take a more active role. See Tip #96 for more ideas.

THE CHANGE: She might be uncomfortable and unsure of herself in her New Mom Thong.
THE ACTION PLAN: Give her permission to be tired, hormonal, overwhelmed, emotional, irritable, and unsure of herself. Encourage her to put together a plan ahead of time—she's going to need a support system. If she doesn't have friends or family, help her find support. Connect her with other moms or professional care (see Tip #42).

THE CHANGE: You might feel financial stress.

THE ACTION PLAN: Evaluate your finances months before the baby arrives. Figure out how much things will cost and plan for the months ahead. Don't wait until you're exhausted, stressed, and overwhelmed. That's when fights happen. If you need to get a coach to help you better define your goals, then make that investment. If you have an action plan in place, you'll be focused and on track once change happens. This can mean moving, cutting expenses, or taking on extra work. See Tip #60 for more ideas.

THE CHANGE: You will be sleep-deprived.
THE ACTION PLAN: Craft a sleep strategy before you get home that will help you and your partner get more rest. Check out Tip #97 for more information.

THE CHANGE: You may be unsure of whether or not you're ready to be a dad.
THE ACTION PLAN: The paternal instinct will kick in. When that switch flips on is unpredictable, but it will. Be patient and give yourself permission to take time. Talk to other guys and reach out in the www.DadsPregnant.com discussion forums. See Tip #96 for more info.

No one told us that it was going to be this much fun. Most people told us how hard it would be or how little sleep we're going to get—and all of that is true, but it's just so much fun. We love having our little guy around.
—*Mike (son 4 months)*

THE CHANGE: Your marriage and sex life may change.
THE ACTION PLAN: If you're worried about the relationship changing, talk to

your partner about it and plan how you'll stay connected. Talk to friends or family members who have relationships you respect. Consider talking to a therapist. Once she's cleared by the doctor for sex, know that a rested happy woman is more likely to have sex. Plan for how you will help her be well rested. (See Tip #101.)

THE CHANGE: Your partner's identity will shift.

THE ACTION PLAN: This may happen because she's stopped working; because she has less time for herself, her friends, or her interests; or simply because she has this new person in her life. She simply is not the person she was before the baby. Help her come up with an action plan if she's feeling like her life is unfamiliar and overwhelming. Encourage her to talk to her friends who have been through this transition and make sure you're both aware of the challenges. If you know what people trip over, you can create a new path or jump when you see it coming.

THE CHANGE: You can't hang out with friends as much.

THE ACTION PLAN: Remind yourself that this is temporary. Once you can get through the first few months, things will definitely change. What might shock you is that once you have the baby, you might not want to do the things you used to do. You might not be as upset as you thought about missing a night out.

THE CHANGE: You have feelings of overwhelming responsibility.

THE ACTION PLAN: When something feels overwhelming, turn to the people who have done this before you and ask them to put things in perspective. Find out what they did right and what they did wrong. If you don't have family or friends to talk with, then find a therapist to help you deal with this. It will pass, but if your partner isn't available to talk about this and your friends aren't informed, you might need a professional.

THE CHANGE: You're stressed.

THE ACTION PLAN: Compile a list of the healthy outlets you will turn to in order to deal with the stress. Plan on going to the gym and build it into your schedule. Create a way to support your partner and still take care of yourself. Work with your partner and figure out how you can both manage it.

THE CHANGE: No one is sure how to take care of a baby at first.

THE ACTION PLAN: Research and register for a parenting class together. Pick up the book *The Happiest Baby on the Block* by Dr. Harvey Karp. Discuss this with your friends. Practice changing diapers. Taking care of a kid is a hard thing to do. Read ahead together. Make this a project you start before the baby is born. Then, when the kid arrives, you'll have a plan instead of sitting there in the middle of the night wondering what the hell to do next (I'm pointing a finger at me).

THE CHANGE: Fill in the blank at www.Dads Pregnant.com.
THE ACTION PLAN: Fill in the blank at www.Dads Pregnant.com.

THE BOTTOM LINE:
Help men (and women) understand what's coming their way by sharing your tips, stories, and experiences as they unfold (www.DadsPregnant.com). Truly, we are pioneers…

Tip #93
The First Night Home—aka the All-Nighter

THE TIP:
It's not as bad as it initially seems the first two or three days…

THE STORY:
Our daughter stayed in the room with us at the hospital. When she cried, the nurses were right there to help us. Once we lost the nurses' help, we felt overwhelmed at home. When we left the hospital, we were terrified. I remember my wife turning to me and saying, "I can't believe they're letting us leave with this

little baby." When we got home, it was just the two of us. We felt all alone. We didn't think we'd need help so we didn't ask for it. The first night was miserable. Every time we fed our daughter she would fall asleep in our arms. Then we would place her down and she would wake up and cry. This happened over and over again, at least fifty times, all night long. We were telling each other we couldn't do this. We didn't know if we were cut out for it. How could this be so miserable when it was all supposed to be beautiful? The second and third night my mom stayed with us and helped (she would have stayed longer, but we didn't think we'd need her), but it got better. My wife did some research and we became familiar with what our daughter wanted. It took a few nights of practice to figure it out, but we did get her to sleep. It got so much better we decided to have a second daughter. See, it does get better.

—Thad, daughters 11 months and 3 years

✳ ✳ ✳

They didn't give us a manual.

She came with no instructions.

We were just supposed to know what to do with our newborn.

But we had no idea what the hell we were doing.

My wife was exhausted from giving birth. I was exhausted from not sleeping at the hospital. And this little person was exhausted from being evicted from the womb. We were all having our issues.

Our first three nights were spent sitting in bed with our arms crossed and our daughter nestled on our chests (accidental kangaroo care). We propped pillows under our elbows to support our arms while we half-slept. We used our knees and a pillow for additional support. The engineering assured our daughter was safe in our arms as we slept. When we got brave, we'd place her in the co-sleeper next to the bed (a co-sleeper is like a crib that connects to the bed; the sleeping part of the name is highly deceptive). The baby never slept. The only way she would sleep was if she was resting in our arms. We knew this wasn't how it should be. But no one told us how it should be. Was this how it could be? Three nights later, we got smart—actually my wife got smart and turned to the books.

BACK TO SLEEP CAMPAIGN:

If your baby is under twelve months old, you can help reduce the risk of SIDS (Sudden Infant Death Syndrome), suffocation, and strangulation by following these three tips (Source: www.cpsc.gov/):

1. Place your baby to sleep on his or her back. Babies who sleep on their backs have a much lower risk of SIDS and suffocation.
2. Remove all soft bedding from the crib. A baby can suffocate from soft bedding in a crib. Be sure to remove all pillows, quilts, comforters,

BACK TO SLEEP CAMPAIGN: (Contd.)

and sheepskins from your crib.

3. Put your baby to sleep in a safe crib. A safe crib is the best place for your baby to sleep. Make sure your crib has no missing or broken hardware, no slats more than 2 $\frac{3}{8}$ inches apart, no corner posts over $\frac{1}{16}$ inch high, no cutout designs in the head-board or footboard, a firm, tight-fitting mattress, and a safety certification seal (on new cribs).

WHAT IS SIDS?

Sudden Infant Death Syndrome (SIDS) is the

The one that saved us was *The Happiest Baby on the Block* by Dr. Harvey Karp. My wife read the important parts to me at 3:00 a.m. huddled in the bathroom. In the book, Dr. Karp refers to the three months following birth as the fourth trimester. During the fourth trimester, the infant's calming reflex can be stimulated by applying the 5 "S's": 1) swaddling (tight wrapping of the baby) 2) side/stomach (laying baby on her left side or stomach while awake, 3) shushing, 4) swinging, and 5) sucking.

What helped us survive:

- **Swaddling** our daughter kept her tight in the blanket (babies twitch and their body parts can swing around and wake them up). We got good at wrapping her up. The swaddle blankets look confining, but they were awesome.

- **Side/stomach:** Our daughter had bad reflux so holding her on her side and stomach (while she was awake) helped calm her down.
- **Shushing:** When she cried I would shush her again and again. Think of a silence-crazed librarian "shushing" loudly over and over again—that's how you shush.
- **Swinging:** The motion helped calm her down (swings work, our arms worked, anything that swings works).
- **Sucking:** We got her a different kind of pacifier than the one from the hospital and it made all the difference.

BACK TO SLEEP CAMPAIGN: (Contd.) leading cause of death among infants aged 1 to 12 months, and is the third leading cause overall of infant mortality in the United States. Although the overall rate of SIDS in the United States has declined by more than 50% since 1990, rates have declined less among non-Hispanic Black and American Indian/Alaska Native infants. African American babies die from SIDS at more than twice the rate of other babies. Preventing SIDS remains an important public health priority. (source: www.cdc.gov/SIDS/)

The Happiest Baby on the Block is also available on DVD (www.thehappiestbaby.com). Pack a portable DVD player to bring to the hospital and watch it. Put it on your packing list for the delivery. Get a head start and start off the first night with a plan.

A couple more things (although this might be totally useless for you): We used a positioner for sleeping (it lays in the crib and has two little wedges, like bookends, so the baby feels nice and cozy). We also elevated one end of the crib under the feet (the end where her head rested). Of course, ask your caregiver for a list of books and ideas. If you're having a challenging night or two or a hundred, do not hesitate to call your doctor with concerns.

THE BOTTOM LINE:

Newborns don't come with user's manuals, but there are some available. Ask your doctor, friends, and family to offer suggestions. Put them in your backpack to take to the hospital. Watch *The Happiest Baby on the Block* DVD while passing time during labor (then watch the breastfeeding channel).

Tip #94
HELP WANTED: Loving Your In-Laws Like Never Before

THE TIP:
A man needs to remind his mother that she is not the mother's mother, and the relationship between his mom and his wife will never be the same as the relationship between his wife and her mom.

THE STORY:
I knew that my mother-in-law was excited about the grandchild and helping me during my recovery, but when my ass is hurting from giving birth, and I'm the one who is exhausted, I want my mommy there to take care of me, not his. We know she's there and available. We'll call when we need help. And it's his job to run interference if his mother is overbearing. (P.S. I love my mother-in-law—she's an excellent grandmother!)

—*Misti, daughter 2 years*

✳ ✳ ✳

- If someone offers help, take them up on it.
- If someone offers to bring you dinner, accept it.

My mother-in-law helped us out with our newborn daughter. When she left, that was the saddest I've ever been to see my mother-in-law leave.
—*Thad (daughters 11 months and 3 years)*

- If someone offers to pay for a night nurse as a gift, let them.
- If your mom or mother-in-law offers to spend a week with you, let her.
- If your mom or mother in-law offers to spend two weeks with you, let her.
- If your partner is overwhelmed, hire help (if financially possible).
- If your partner is depressed, help her find help (see Tip #49).

Take advantage of all the help you can get. Sure you might like the idea of spending time together as a family, but you have your entire life to be a family. Yes, there will be times when a house guest will wear out her welcome. There will be moments when you think it was a big mistake, but the bigger mistake is not letting people help. Even the most annoying, obnoxious, and irritating family can be helpful. You just need to set boundaries and know that it's only temporary. Take all the help offered.

Giving birth and caring for a newborn is exhausting. Don't be a hero and tell everyone that you'll manage. Unless you manage an infant day care and are used to caring for newborns, you'll discover that newborns need constant care and attention. After the first few weeks, you'll wish you had some help. Get help sooner rather than later.

Don't refuse help. Even if someone wants to hold the baby for a few minutes, take them up on it.

—*Jeff (daughter 9 months, son 5½ years)*

I thought we could do it on our own—and the truth is that we survived, but I wasn't the one getting up three times a night to nurse for thirty to forty-five minutes. I wasn't the one who gave birth or managed the baby's sleeping, eating, clothing, and care. She needs as much help as possible—from you, from friends, from family, from paid professionals. The rest of this chapter mentions other things you can do to help, so plan on helping. The little things will make a profound difference.

When someone asks you the question, "What can I do to help?" ask them to send dinner (this implies that they will not be joining you). She's not going to want to cook and you're not going to want to cook. It's a luxury when meals are ready to cook or prepared for you. If someone wants to do something very special and they have a budget, ask about a night nurse. A night nurse is great because she will bring the baby to your partner (if breastfeeding) and allow her and you to stay in bed and feed. When it comes to things like cleaning the house, it might be worth hiring a service to come once every few weeks or so—this is something you can build into your budget.

WARNING: Postpartum women are still hormonal. In fact, postpartum hormones can be even more intense and powerful. The physical and emotional changes coupled with the hormonal surge can mean that your partner might say

> Shield her from constant visitors all day; only let people in who are going to help you and not tire you out by expecting you to entertain them.
>
> —*Elizabeth (daughter 7 months)*

or do things that will aggravate or annoy you. This can be even more challenging to navigate when you're overtired and overwhelmed. The hormones will wane, but until then allow her to be right even when she's wrong. Help her through this by allowing her to ride the hormonal highway. If at any time you think she might be suffering from postpartum depression (PPD), let her doctor know and insist she get help (see Tip #49).

THE BOTTOM LINE:
There's no such thing as being too helpful.

Tip #95
NURSING AND BOTTLE-FEEDING: Supporting Her Milky Breasts and Using a Bottle

THE TIP:
If she's breastfeeding, the onus is on her to feed your baby—no one else can do it, and that is a heavy responsibility when you're overtired.

THE STORY:
He helped me succeed because he never made negative comments; he took her downstairs when she was unsettled so I could sleep and brought her up for a feed. New babies always seem to want to be fed when your food is ready, so he often fed me while I nursed. I

was also always thirsty but initially needed two hands to feed. I discovered that he is also an expert at holding a glass so I could drink without spilling down my front. Our families also took over the household tasks for me for the first three weeks. A man shouldn't underestimate how invaluable those small things are. I couldn't have done it without his help, and yet at the time they seemed like such simple things to do.

—Elizabeth, daughter 7 months

✸ ✸ ✸

Either your baby will be on formula, breast milk, or a combination of the two.

When I was born, formula was the fashionable way to feed a baby. The trend has shifted back to mother's milk. My wife nursed for about ten months. It was all-consuming at times. It was stressful to watch her go through it. With the baby feeding every two to three hours, she was constantly pumping, waking up, and whipping it out (her breast—and more like gently pulling it out).

The big questions a new mom has on her mind before birth: Will I produce milk? Will the baby latch on? Will I produce enough milk for my baby? All of these things can weigh heavily on your partner and build up

I think of breastfeeding as the biggest accomplishment of my life—bigger than college, bigger than grad school, or anything I've done in my career.

—Stephanie (daughter 23 months, 25 weeks pregnant)

expectations. And the overwhelming message from a large part of the medical community is "breastfeeding is best."

Personally, I preferred that she did whatever worked for her. As a formula-fed baby with a tobacco-scented amniotic sac (my mom was a pregnant smoker before there were warning labels), I like to use my own experience as the litmus test. Therefore, I didn't pressure her one way or the other. I liked the idea of breast milk because it can save a lot of money (formula is expensive). I didn't factor in the emotional, physical, and logistical aspects of being married to a nursing woman. Seriously, her world centered around her breasts and the baby's feeding schedule.

A LOOK AT MILKY BREASTS

Milky breasts are remarkable. What's so incredible is that my wife's breasts would regulate their own milk production based on my daughter's intake. If my daughter didn't feed for a while, my wife's breasts would become engorged and swell up to an inhuman size—think the fakest biggest breasts at a rural strip club (no disrespect to my wife's breasts or rural strip clubs). When she saw a picture of my daughter or heard my

> No one told me that I would get engorged and sore and that it would be a really awkward process for the first week or so. It's not only hard physically, it's also hard emotionally.
> —*Maggie (son 3 months)*

> Breastfeeding is great for some women, but not all. The most important thing is getting sleep and having a happy wife.
> —*Cathy (sons 4 months and 3½ years)*

daughter's cry, her milk would "let down." Let down is the equivalent of the dam breaking—she was ready to flow. Let down could also mean leaking, spritzing, or spraying milk.

Those breasts were really quite amazing. Because my wife was working, she had to do a lot of pumping. She needed to pump to keep up her milk production and to have enough milk for our daughter when she was at work. We were always talking about her milk production. She was like a dairy farmer. She would then take the milk and freeze it. (A side note: Once, the freezer broke, and she lost about 45 ounces of breast milk. She literally was crying over spilled thawed milk.)

Getting a good night's sleep the first six weeks for her meant getting three hours of uninterrupted sleep. When she did nightly feedings, it wasn't like the baby would chug the milk. She was averaging about thirty minutes a feeding. Then she had to change the diaper and soothe our daughter. Between getting up, feeding the baby, and getting her back down, it was exhausting. This is true of all moms who get up to do feedings—not just nursing moms. The most helpful thing a man can do is to bring the baby to her in the middle of the night and put the baby back down. If he can do the feeding too, that's even more helpful.

WAYS TO SUPPORT HER AND HER BREASTS

Get an Expert Involved: She might not know how her milk-making breasts work. Suggest that she get the name of a lactation consultant before she walks into

WHY BREASTFEED YOUR BABY?

1. A mother's milk has just the right amount of fat, sugar, water, and protein that is needed for a baby's growth and development. Most babies find it easier to digest breast milk than formula. Breast milk contains agents (called antibodies) that help protect infants from bacteria and viruses and help them fight off infection and disease. Human milk straight from the breast is always sterile.

2. Breastfeeding saves time and money. You do not have to purchase, measure, the hospital. Also, before the baby is born, see if there's a lactation consultant at the hospital. If she should have questions or a problem, turn her breasts in the direction of a consultant. Sometimes the consultation can be covered under insurance (talk to your pediatrician or caregiver).

Respect Her Choice: Don't pressure her to nurse if she's not interested. Breastfeeding takes an unwavering commitment. If she's not up for it, don't force her (although I don't think you could force her because they're her breasts).

Not All Women Produce Enough: Until she gives birth she won't know if she can produce milk. Even if she can produce milk, it might not be enough milk. Do not put pressure on her to nurse. If she is unable to produce enough milk, pressuring her will only make her feel like she disappointed you. She'll have a hard enough time dealing with it herself.

Bring the Baby to Her: Getting up at night and putting the baby down can take time. Even if you're working and she's working, figure out how you can help.

Bring Water to Her: She needs to stay hydrated and nourished. Get her a special mug or water bottle to help her keep up her water intake.

Buy a Breast Pump: If she's up for pumping, get a quality breast pump. There are hand breast pumps, but I imagine you would probably cramp up after an ounce or two. Electric ones are most efficient. If she can pump, then she can put some milk in a bottle and you can enjoy feeding your baby too. Gift idea: Pimp up her pump with rhinestones for Mother's Day…

WHY BREASTFEED YOUR BABY? (Contd.)

and mix formula, and there are no bottles to warm in the middle of the night.

3. Breastfeeding also helps a mother bond with her baby. Physical contact is important to newborns and can help them feel more secure, warm, and comforted. Nursing uses up extra calories, making it easier to lose the pounds gained from pregnancy. It also helps the uterus get back to its original size more quickly and lessens any bleeding a woman may have after giving birth.

Tasting the Milk: It's kind of like sweet sugar water. I've never had a cup of breast milk or dipped Oreos in

WHY BREASTFEED YOUR BABY? (Contd.)

Breastfeeding also may lower the risk of breast and ovarian cancers.

4. The U.S. Surgeon General recommends that babies be fed with breast milk only—no formula—for the first six months of life. It is better to breastfeed for six months and best to breastfeed for twelve months, or for as long as you and your baby wish. Solid foods can be introduced when the baby is six months old, while you continue to breastfeed. (Source: www.4women.gov)

it, but I did taste it. My wife put a drop in my mouth. I gagged. There's something programmed into our heads that the milk isn't for us.

Her Enormous Milky Breasts: Milk-producing breasts can be huge, but they're better left untouched. When getting back together, consider protective eyewear and pads. Breasts spray, leak, and spritz when you least expect it.

ABOUT BOTTLE-FEEDING

If your baby is on formula or if your nursing partner pumps, you will be lucky enough to feed the baby. Feeding a baby can be intimidating. (Actually, doing anything with a baby can be intimidating.)

I'm fortunate enough to live with a feeding expert. It's not that she's an expert at feeding herself (no feeding jokes—remember, she's pregnant); my wife is a specialist in infant feeding and swallowing. She spends her time working in a rehabilitation hospital, private practice, and a NICU helping infants and children become better eaters. Having an expert with me was so helpful when feeding and choosing the right bottle for our daughter. My wife showed me how to hold the baby, how to hold the bottle, and how the different nipples can control the flow. It's hard to know what kind of flow, nipple, and bottle will work. No one is expecting you to know, but if your partner gets frustrated, know that there are options. Feeding can be a source of stress, whether it's by bottle or nursing. If you have any issues, talk to your pediatrician and or a specialist. There are also community websites for new moms with some very active discussion boards.

SUGGESTING READING:
Child of Mine: Feeding with Love and Good Sense by Ellyn Satter

If your partner is nursing and you would like to help with the feeding, ask if she can pump so you can help. If she's not comfortable pumping, bring the baby over to her to feed and then put the baby back to sleep. If

BREASTFEEDING BOOKS:

Encourage her to only read books that are recommended by a lactation consultant, doctor, or a friend who shares a similar philosophy. Some issues relating to childbirth can evoke strong emotions. Breastfeeding is one of those issues.

the baby is formula-fed, build up your confidence early and do some feedings in the hospital when the nursing staff is available. Your style can be different than her style but still be a good style. When it comes to feeding the baby, here are the top five things you should avoid:

- Forcing a bottle in a baby's mouth when he's not taking it readily.
- Jiggling a bottle in a baby's mouth to keep her sucking.
- Trying to keep feeding a baby who is giving you signals he is all done.
- Ignoring repeated signs of trouble with feeding: frequent coughing, gagging, excessive spitting up, formula coming out the baby's nose.
- Thinking you can't feed the baby the right way—you can develop your own style; just because you do it differently doesn't mean it's wrong.

THE BOTTOM LINE:

If you pump your breasts as a gesture of support, make sure to clean the hoses thoroughly before she uses the pump again.

Tip #96
TAKE A SHIFT A WEEK: Getting Peed On, Pooped On, and Helping Out…

THE TIP:

If she's at home during the week and you're working during the week, take care of the baby at least one day on the weekend. It will give your wife time to take care of herself and find some balance—she needs it.

THE STORY:

It's hard for men to understand that taking care of a newborn can be all-consuming. It's hard to get things done. My husband would come home from work and say he's going to get a haircut, going to the cleaners, and going to exercise. And I'm like, "I've needed to do that for the last three months." Men can pick up and go whenever they want. Work obligations are work obligations, but when they're not working, it's nice when they take over. My husband didn't realize how hard it was for me to get things done until I talked to him about it. On the weekends, he'll be in charge of our son for a whole Sunday. He tells me which nights he'll be home and what's happening on the weekend in advance. Some nights, I'll go out and run my errands. So he understands. Some of my friends have told me that the only way men will understand is if you leave them alone with the kid for the entire week. Sometimes, after a long day, I want nothing to do with my son. I'm like, you feed him, you give him dinner, you read him stories—I just don't want anything to do with him, but I still love him.

—Tami, son 18 months, pregnant with #2

✳ ✳ ✳

A baby-sitter is technically someone who gets paid (unless he or she is family) to take care of the baby while the parents are away. Therefore, a dad isn't a baby-sitter (although it might feel like it the first time). Being left alone in a room with your newborn might freak you out. It's hard to know how a baby works. While it's intimidating to think that you are in charge for a day, there's nothing like being the one in control. There are a few reasons why you should do this:

- It's one thing to hear about it, but to live it will give you a completely different perspective. Feeding the baby, changing the baby, putting the baby down for a

I've had every bodily fluid on me—poop, pee, vomit, and diarrhea. It's a rite of passage all dads experience.
—Eliot (father of two)

nap, playing with the baby, and taking care of the baby all day long is a lot of work—physically and emotionally. If you have a baby who screams, it's that much more exhausting. One afternoon was all it took for me to understand—thank God for Elmo (he helped my daughter chill out when she lost it for forty-five minutes)!

- Give your partner time to find some balance in her life. Taking care of a newborn is exhausting. As one dad said, "It's not 24/7, it's 24/7/10,080 (the 10,080 are the minutes that make up the week)." If she's nursing, she's that much more tied to the baby. If you want her to be happy, which is essential for having a happy home, which is essential for your happiness, then she needs to find some balance. She needs time to work out, get her hair and nails done, take a nap, hang out with friends without the baby, and take a little time to renew, refresh, and get reinvigorated. Give a little, and you'll get so much back.

- Take the time to bond with the baby. There's something to be said about doing things the way you want. I'm not saying you should make up your own rules and violate the sleeping schedule, but you don't have to worry about doing something wrong when she's not around. Also, you can learn how

> I never minded changing my son's diaper. With my daughter, I'm afraid of hurting her and you don't know how it all works—it can be a little intimidating.
>
> —Mark (son 2½ years, daughter 10 months)

to operate your baby without a safety net. If you're lucky, while you're taking care of the baby he or she might cry, spit up, vomit, pee, poop, or have diarrhea on you—handling all the little things on your own will help you feel more confident and connected. And the best part: one day you can tell your daughter or son all about it.

THE BOTTOM LINE:
I've been peed on, projectile vomited on, and diarrhea-ed on—and I can't wait to talk about it at her wedding toast. Cheers!

Tip #97
SLEEPING AND NOT SLEEPING: Crafting a Sleep Strategy before Getting Sleepy

THE TIP:
A man should realize that mom needs time to get healthy and heal, otherwise recovery is going to be a lot longer.

THE STORY:
Our first daughter was colicky and cried for hours on end. It was very overwhelming for us. She wouldn't stop crying. She was high-maintenance since day one and still is. We had a hard time settling whose turn it was to hold her and who gets out of the house. We

ended up taking turns at night when it came to sleeping. I would get the first half of the night to sleep and he would get the second half of the night. At least we would each get about five straight hours. Our second two were angels because we weren't so tense. He was very helpful with all three and it made it manageable.

—Joann, daughters 2 years (twins) and 4 years

✳ ✳ ✳

Let's start with the basics:
- A newborn will sleep roughly 16 hours a day.
- Sleep will be in 2- to 4-hour stretches at a time.
- Figure that a feeding takes 30 to 45 minutes.
- For every 8 hours of uninterrupted sleep you get, she may sleep for a total of 5 to 6 interrupted hours (this is factoring in three feedings and changing and soothing the baby back to sleep after each feeding).

All this sleeping will screw up your schedule. Newborns will nap more than a kid home from college during winter break. They have about sixty minutes of awake time and then they sleep. It's a little ridiculous.

The biggest challenge was SLEEP—for us and the baby. I was so naive. I honestly thought that the baby would only wake up once a night because I only woke up once a night during my pregnancy.

—Megan (daughter 11 months)

I fought this early on, and it caused a lot of problems. Having sixty minutes of awake time meant that we didn't have a lot of time to go out and do things. Some moms don't mind if a baby sleeps in the car seat, but other moms want the baby home in the crib (it all depends on what sleep training method you follow—yes, there are training methods). My wife was 100 percent right, but I never took the time to read the sleep training books. Instead, I just resisted the method. As a result, I turned my wife into the bad guy when she would insist on putting our daughter down for nap time. I still feel bad that I put her in that position.

This sleep thing will be a big deal. Do yourself a favor and either play an active role in researching methods with her or respect her way of running the show. And then, when you're out with grandparents and they want to push the baby a little later, instead of letting her take the heat, explain that loving their grandchild should mean wanting their grandchild to get a good night's sleep and not be overtired and cranky the next morning.

You would think with the baby sleeping so much, you would get a lot of sleep, but newborns are unpredictable sleepers. A colicky baby or a newborn with excessive reflux can cry for hours and hours at a time (those are the wakeful hours). You won't know what kind

The sleep deprivation is something I'm used to because of my work in higher ed. It was good for us because she could rest in the morning and I'd get up with the kids.

—*Craig (sons 7 months and 2½ years)*

of baby you have until you meet him or her, but in the meantime you can prepare for what's ahead.

Talk to a hundred guys and ask them if they had a sleep strategy when they came home, and they'll tell you that they were lucky to remember the car seat. Devising a sleep strategy is not something most of us think about ahead of time—mainly because no one tells us we should.

All anyone tells us is how tired we will be when the baby gets here. They don't tell us how to avoid being tired. You are not going to get as much sleep as you got before the baby arrived, but you can get more sleep than the guys complaining about it if you do some planning. Without a plan you can plan on being sleep-deprived.

Sleep is hard to come by the first few months (it will get better). But there is sleep to be had. There is a way to make this work, or at least pretend that it can work. Until you know if you have a good sleeper, it's hard to know if you'll get some good sleeping in. Before you leave the hospital (or wherever you have this baby), develop a sleep strategy. Talk to friends, family, your doctor, or midwife.

Here are some strategies that may help you find some sleep:

- Take as much time off as you can from work during the first couple of weeks and help her to heal so she can get her strength back.

  I was so sleep-deprived I drove away after pumping gas with the nozzle still in the gas tank of my car.

  —*Gary (sons 3 years and 6 months)*

- You need to figure out how the baby works so that you can get comfortable helping her out during the first week or two.
- Whoever is working gets to sleep during the week. Whoever is working as the primary caregiver does weeknight feedings. If the working partner can help during weeknights and still be functional, even better.
- On the weekends, whoever was working does the nighttime feedings. If that's not possible because your partner is nursing, this means helping her by bringing the baby to her (so she can get more sleep), and it means giving her time to nap during the weekend.
- The rule: Caregivers nap when the baby is napping (as long as you're not out shopping—do not nap in department stores).
- Sleep in shifts or sleep in separate rooms. There's no reason for two people to be exhausted. Over the weekend, it will be her turn to sleep in (assuming she's on maternity leave).
- Once one of you returns to work, if sleep is an issue, consider getting a night nurse once a week for a few weeks. If two sets of grandparents are available, have one set help out the first week and the other help the second week. Then rotate them back through until you can handle it on your own.
- Get some sleep books and read them. Swaddling, soothing, and kangaroo care are a few strategies

that can help. Gather techniques and ideas from friends, family, and the pros so you're ready before you need it.

- Read the sleeping techniques in Tip #93 and *The Happiest Baby on the Block*—that book saved our lives.
- Talk to your pediatrician or family doctor. Sometimes kids who can't sleep could be having other issues. They might be able to offer you some suggestions that will make this transition easier.

INSIGHT INTO THE FAMILY BED

(**Author note:** The CDC does not promote a family bed, citing increased risk of SIDS.)

My wife and I never decided to have a family bed, it just happened. We started out like most families—a small crib next to our queen-sized bed. When our daughter would cry in the middle of the night because of hunger, it was easiest for my wife to wake up and nurse. Over time, this routine became more comfortable. Sydney grew larger, and the fear of crushing her in her sleep slowly faded. I can remember a couple of times Sydney kicking me to get me off of her. That is when I became comfortable with having her in our bed. This routine hasn't changed yet; Sydney is now 18 months and still wants to nurse in the middle of the night. My wife is so comfortable with this routine that she doesn't necessarily wake up to nurse. We were both in agreement about this. Other people certainly think we are strange, but they have gotten used to the idea. I don't really care too much about other people's opinions on this matter. The setup has certainly affected our sex life. I know that our parents would like our daughter to sleep in her own bed because they think we need to have another child. It's actually made us more romantic when we have had the bed to ourselves. We actually had to have sex dates. We have taken our daughter over to grandma's house and come home for a couple of hours just so that we could have sex. Nothing wrong with that!

—Jeff, daughter 18 months

THE BOTTOM LINE:
Don't stay up too late creating your sleep strategy.

Tip #98
WORKING AT HOME: Setting Up a Conference Call during Nap Time

THE TIP:
It might not work out according to the plan. It may take time to figure it out.

THE STORY:

My wife works full time and I work from a home office half the year. The plan was for her to work from home on Fridays and take care of him while getting work done. The expectation was that I would also help watch the baby while trying to get work done. It turned out that neither one of us could get anything done. Between feeding him and playing with him, it was impossible. One Friday, she was out running some errands while I was working at home. I had a conference call scheduled during his nap time. Well, that day he woke up early from his morning nap hungry and crying. I also needed to take this call. The only way I could keep him quiet was to feed him during the conference call. I was staring at him in the eyes begging him not to cry. I'm sure the people on the call heard some feeding baby noises, but there wasn't anything else I could do. After this incident, I pretty much told my wife that I can't take care of him and work. She couldn't get anything done either and respected it. We made adjustments. Now, on Fridays, we drop off our son at her parents' house after playing and eating breakfast in the morning. It took a while to figure out how to make it work.

—Irl, son 22 months, 28 weeks pregnant

✳ ✳ ✳

She comes home with the groceries and I help put away the groceries. Then I play with my son. And before I know it, I've been away from work for three hours.

—Matt (sons 1 month and 2½ years)

Working at home becomes an entirely new experience when you have a baby at home. The problem is if you are supposed to be working at home and don't get your work done at home, you risk not having a job or a home—which makes working at home that much more difficult. Some suggestions for how to not lose your job and house:

SET BOUNDARIES

You will become your own worst enemy. There will be times you want to take a break and play with your newborn. Before you know it, you'll be changing a diaper, soothing a crying baby, preparing a bottle, putting together a new toy, and jumping around like an idiot. Then the phone will ring and you'll remember that you're supposed to be at work. Unless you work in day care or at a studio that records baby sound effects, it's better to let the call go to voicemail.

The next problem is that your partner will distract you (even if she's not trying to). Having you around means that you're, well, around. And being accessible means that it's easy to call out to you when a cute thing happens, or when she needs more diapers, or when you need to bring up clothes, make a bottle, or help during a crisis. Being at home with a sick kid... well, forget it—not getting called into a vomit or explosive poop episode is impossible. Setting boundaries can be a challenge.

DISCUSS ERRANDS AND APPOINTMENTS

If your partner is on maternity leave, having her home will take up some of your time. She might want to run an errand, get her hair cut, or have lunch with a friend. She might schedule a service call or some kind of delivery. She might want to run out to the gym for an hour. Discuss this with her ahead of time and work out a system. Otherwise when she has a doctor's appointment, you will find yourself putting the baby down for a nap at the same time you have a conference call planned.

GET OUT OF THE HOUSE

Go to a coffee house or a restaurant with wireless Internet connection. These days you can pretty much take your computer and go online almost anywhere. I know because I've been everywhere. There's always a place to go. Sometimes, that's what you need.

STRUCTURE THE DAY

Have breakfast together, have lunch together, and set a quitting time. It might vary, but if your partner knows that you have structure, she can check with you first when she needs you to do something during the day, or she can save it for later. The structure is as much for you as it is for those sharing the house and space with you.

FORWARD A BIZ CALL TO CELL

The secret is to work at home and never have anyone know that you're working at home. If you're on the phone with a client, the baby screaming and the dog barking won't do anything to help you close the deal—unless you're supposed to be working at a kennel or day care facility. Make sure you use your cell phone as your primary line or have your business line forward to your cell phone during noisy times. This way you can always leave the room if someone or something gets too noisy.

GET AN OFFICE

I know you don't want to take on the expense of an office after taking on the expense of a baby, but sometimes being home can reduce productivity to the point that the expense of moving out becomes an investment to increase productivity. Keep the thought at the back of your mind. You might be increasing expenses, but you'll ultimately increase revenue.

THE BOTTOM LINE:

You can have breakfast, lunch, and dinner with your new family and still be able to pay for breakfast, lunch, and dinner working from home.

Tip #99
The Stay-at-Home Dad—aka the Do-It-All Dad

THE TIP:
Your wife and friends will be jealous.

THE STORY:
I decided to stay at home because my wife now makes about seven times what I was making, and she travels a lot for work. I hated my job and waited until they fired me (to get unemployment) which was about a month before the second baby was born. My responsibilities are to the kids and the house (and dog). I don't have clients who need things. My older son and I can play sports and video games together. My wife is jealous, because she wanted to be the stay-at-home mom. I told her to quit; we'd move to a smaller house, and stop vacations, dinners, etc. She'd rather have the money. My friends are jealous. I call them during the day to ask if they can go to an early afternoon baseball game or to the race track, and they are busy at work (I have a sitter come in once a week). When the baby sleeps, then I can read, play on the computer, or go to sleep. I went to the first PTA meeting of the year. Out of forty-three people, I was the only man. On school field trips, I'm the only dad. Most moms think it's great (at least

Those years of staying at home are precious to me and a privilege that most men don't get.

—*David (father of two)*

that's what they tell me) that I stay home with the kids. All that matters is what my wife thinks. The one thing they don't understand is that when the baby is not sleeping, I'm not sleeping. This week the kids have been sick, and I've been suffering from major sleep deprivation. I must admit, I do enjoy that some of my male friends are jealous.

—Jeff, daughter 7 months, son 5 years

✳ ✳ ✳

The idea of being a stay-at-home dad might have never even crossed your mind until reading this. You might be thinking you'd love to do this, but you don't want to "stay at home." However stay-at-home dads are allowed to go out and do a lot of things. They can go shopping, go to the park, and go to sporting events in the afternoon (if you get a sitter).

Given that 33 percent of the workforce is working at home, a lot of full-time workers are part-time stay-at-home dads and don't even know it. I don't even think they realize it. Their employers don't realize it either, but fathers' roles are constantly shifting. With the Internet, cell phones, and laptops, you can work during nap times, while waiting in the car during carpools, or after bedtime. For couples who work different shifts (mom works days and dad works nights), the father is playing a larger role. Then there are dads who are the primary caregivers over the weekend. The reality is that the line between the working-outside-the-home dad and the stay-at-home dad has been so blurred that it's time for a new expression. I just don't think the term stay-at-home dad is appropriate anymore. How about a do-it-all dad? That seems much more appropriate.

Given the significant role we play in the pregnancy experience, it's not surprising that more men are sticking around and wanting to stick around. Do-it-all dads (formerly known as stay-at-home dads) can find support groups, conventions, forums, and organizations where they can share information with other dads. Whether the choice is made for financial reasons or personal reasons, I've never met a guy who has said it sucked. I'm sure there are some out there (it's nice to meet you all) who don't like it, but it's not a bad life. As technology makes us

TRENDS:
Working at home (from The Department of Education)

In a dramatic contrast to the changes stimulated by the industrial revolution, which drove workers out of the home and into the factory, the current technological revolution has created an opportunity for the return of market work to the home. Recent sample surveys conducted by Link Resources Corporation report that the number of people who do some of the work for their primary jobs at home grew, on average, 8.9 percent annually between 1989 and 1993; by the latter year, 33.0 percent of the adult work force engaged in some work at home.
http://stats.bls.gov/opub/mlr/1996/11/art3exc.htm

more independent and mobile, I wouldn't be surprised to see fathers working shorter weeks or perhaps shifting their work hours to after bedtime and spending more time with their kids. There's no shame in being actively involved and engaged in your child's life. I think it's cool.

THE BOTTOM LINE:
The "do-it-all dad"—the man who plays every role. Have a better name to replace the term stay-at-home dad? Send it to me via www.DadsPregnant.com.

Tip #100
WORKING ON THE ROAD: Being There When You're Not Really There...

THE TIP:
When on the road, take advantage of technology to help you stay connected.

THE STORY:
I'm probably on the road over a hundred days a year. One of the things we've been doing to help deal with it is video conferencing. A few months after the baby was born, we got two Mac laptops. It's a made a huge difference. I kind of know the baby's nap schedule, so if it's before 9:26 a.m. Nashville time, I can tell my

wife I'm online. She'll turn on the computer and then I'll play with my daughter. We'll wave to each other and play peekaboo. I'll bounce from bed to bed making her giggle. It's a strange way of doing it, but I get to play with my baby. When I log off, I'm all alone in my hotel room, and that's kind of weird. We use technology to make it work with me being on the road. It also helps me to stay more connected with my wife. There will be times when I can chat with her for an hour and a half. We'll talk about stuff that we need to figure out—finances, the baby, her new business, and other issues. I can be supportive of her. Of course, it's no substitution for being a husband or father who is home all the time, but it's been great to interact this way when I'm away.

—Jason, daughter 12 months

✳ ✳ ✳

When my oldest brother was born (I have two older brothers), my dad dropped off my mom on the way back from the hospital and hit the road to go on sales calls. He was on the road a few nights a week (selling insurance). He didn't want to be away, but he had to go back to work with a newborn on the payroll and a wife who was no longer working.

I do a lot of speaking events and traveling. I love my job, but I don't love being away from the people I love the most in life.

—Harlan (daughter 22 months, 21 weeks pregnant)

Checking in on the phone meant finding a phone booth or calling from a Howard Johnson's Hotel (he loved the HoJos). Calling from a hotel meant that he could only talk for a few minutes because it was so expensive.

Fast forward thirty-five years and we now have cell phones with free minutes, video phones, online cameras, texting, and free hotel phones—it's the closest thing to being there without physically being there. Because of advances in technology, working on the road doesn't mean being as far away. A live cam or cell phone call isn't the same as being there in person, but they provide ways to stay more connected than ever before.

We're very lucky.

But not being there means that you can't help out. You can't support her during a 3:00 a.m. feeding, you can't soothe the baby when she's crying for three hours, and you can't be there to watch the baby while your partner runs out for a second.

The most important thing to do if you travel a lot is to make sure she has support. When you're away, she's not going to have a break. In addition to being there online and on the phone for her, it's important that she has someone else available at home when you're away for long periods of time. This could mean encouraging her to have a sitter a couple times a week so she can get things done. Ask your family and friends to check in with her and drop by when you're not around. If you don't know a lot of people, make an effort through work friends to connect her with people with whom she has something in common. If you don't live near family, it could mean thinking about a possible move so that she can find support while you're gone. Also, encourage her to reach out and see if there are new mom groups, playgroups, or groups where she can meet people with whom she shares common interests.

When you get home from being on the road, as exhausted as you might be, recognize that she's going to need some help. Offer to take the baby for the day or a few hours and encourage her to do whatever she wants to do so she can have time for herself. It's not that she can't take care of the baby, it's just that being a mom 24/7 and not being able to have balance can leave her feeling like she's going out of her mind. I do a lot of speaking events and traveling. I love my job, but I don't love being away from the people whom I love the most in life. I was fortunate enough to meet a woman whose dad had been on the road her entire life. I asked her the question "Is it hard having a dad who travels so much?" She replies, "People ask me that question a lot. I have to tell you, it's the best. I have friends who have dads who work 40 hours a week at home and they don't ever talk. When my dad is home, he's really home. We do things. We talk. I wouldn't trade that for anything." I thanked her. She had no idea how much that meant to me.

THE BOTTOM LINE:
No matter how many miles away, dads can be closer to home than ever before.

Tip #101
HAVING SEX AGAIN (WITH HER): The Sexual
Hibernation Is Over

THE TIP:
Typically post-baby moms are very happy to wait past 6 weeks. Some women schedule their appointment at 7 weeks to give them extra time.

THE STORY:
I wasn't looking forward to having sex again following the birth, physically or emotionally. It was intimidating and the furthest thing from my mind. The first time we had sex it was like sandpaper; it was dry and it hurt. It took probably a good three or four months for it to not hurt. I wanted to be close to my husband and get past the pain, but for a while kind of dreaded the experience. All my estrogen was going toward breastfeeding and not sex. When I stopped nursing, the sexual desire came back to me and I was finally interested in sex again. I found my husband attractive again. I remember I actually felt a crush on my trainer one week and I was like "MEN MEN—yay, my hormones are back." Be gentle, be patient, don't pester her, and go slow; it can be a traumatic experience.

—Courtney, sons 6 weeks, 29 months

* * *

Before you know it, the time will come for her to have her six-week checkup—also known as the "sex week checkup." Our doctor recommended waiting the standard six weeks, but not all caregivers will offer the same advice.

The six-week checkup is generally when the doctor will check her out and give her the "all clear" or the "not clear" for you to get back to business. Before you take a running start from across the bedroom, know that the doctor doesn't control her vagina. She's still in charge of it. Even if she gets the all clear, she might not be ready for you yet. It might be weeks or even months. Whatever you do, don't take it personally. I know, it's easy to think that you've been patient and you deserve this, but in her eyes, she deserves to sleep and relax. At six weeks she might be exhausted, overwhelmed, and stressed out. She might feel uncomfortable with her body. She might be self-conscious of how it will feel (fearing that you will never want to have sex with her again). She could be worried about pain if she had tearing, dryness, an episiotomy, or a difficult labor. The idea of something stretching her out after all that she's been through might not be a turn-on.

Start slow, keep your expectations to a minimum, and see where that takes you (turn to Tip #57). Be patient and don't pressure her. It could be weeks or months until she's up for the sexual energy you've been building

If your wife is a stay-at-home mom, it will be a while before she is affectionate again. Give her a little alone time and she may be more responsive to your touch.

—*Misti (daughter 2 years)*

If you can't get past the image of her BV burned into your mind, focus on the SV (see pg. 50). It might take a few weeks, but it will all come back to you.

up for the past few months. The better-rested, more comfortable, and more relaxed she feels, the better your chances of reawakening your sexual beast from its deep hibernation.

Once she's ready to resume activity, it's a good idea to have lubrication on hand, especially if she's breastfeeding. Women who are breastfeeding may have dryness. Go slowly and listen to her closely. Let her set the pace. She might feel some discomfort. She might be sensitive. Even if she doesn't feel discomfort, the idea of sex after delivering vaginally can be an emotional hurdle.

If you find that you've gone a long period of time and she's still not comfortable, consider talking to a couples' therapist together. Find someone who specializes in postpartum intimacy issues and work through it together.

Once your sex life starts up again, know that she can get pregnant. There's a misconception that women who breastfeed can't get pregnant. NOT TRUE. Women who are breastfeeding can get pregnant. Unless you want to be flipping back to page one in a few weeks, you need to use some kind of birth control.

THE BOTTOM LINE:
The first time back isn't sex—it's called making love. Tell her that and see if she gets in the mood…

Tip #102
DATING YOUR PREGNANT PARTNER AGAIN: Back to How This All Started

THE TIP:
We are a family, but we will always be a couple.

THE STORY:
I've seen how it works with empty nesters. Once the kids have gone the focus turns back to each other, and unfortunately, when that focus turns back, you may find that you don't have a lot in common, which leads to problems. We try to combat this by having a date night—we go to a movie, go to dinner, and just get away. It's hard to do because I work more hours a week than I can even tell you. She works in finance so tax season is crazy for her. And we have two kids. We're lucky we have family close by, and I have

students I can trust. The whole experience of being part of the labor and delivery and having two kids has shown me a different side of my wife that makes us even closer. Being a couple is something that we always work on because we know it's something we always want to work.

—Craig, sons 7 months and 2½ years

✴ ✴ ✴

Once upon a time you took someone on a date. You were her #1. Then she got pregnant and you moved down one rung on the ladder of importance to #2. When the baby was born you fell to #3.

It's nothing you've done wrong. She has a lot on her mind. Going on a date with you is lost somewhere in the middle of caring for the baby, caring for herself, sleeping, eating, feeding the baby, showering, pumping (if nursing), grocery shopping, managing the house, working, working out, working out the baby's sleep schedule (with you), and adjusting to the role of being a mom.

Weekends are no longer about deciding which restaurant to go to or what movie to see—it's about catching up on sleep and taking care of the bare essentials. While her world is a whirlwind, you've got a long list of issues running through your mind (see Tip #92). Everyone is consumed with other things.

On top of this, it's not like you're as physically connected. There isn't any sex happening the first month. Even if she wanted to have sex there's a pretty good chance it's too soon to do it. If she's the social planner, she might be too preoccupied to make plans for a romantic evening out. This means you need to make the date. And with no prospect of getting lucky, the date is solely about spending time together.

For the first time in your relationship, being a couple means making an effort and doing some planning. This idea of having to plan and having to make an effort is one of the most dramatic shifts that happens to a couple once the baby is born. Before you were parents, you could do whatever you wanted whenever you wanted. Last-minute plans were part of the plan. Once you have a child, spending time together as a couple isn't an automatic because there's always a third. Yes, you can take newborns to dinner or lunch and they might sleep, but it's not the same. A date is the two of you. This takes effort and deliberate planning. That's not a bad thing—it's part of being in a relationship. Making time to spend together takes effort.

So, make the effort.

Do whatever you can to plan a date. Have a family member watch the baby or get a sitter for a couple of hours. If she's nursing and has to pump, make it a short date. A date during the first few months following the birth isn't necessarily dinner and a movie. It can be anything as long as you're doing it together.

DON'T TALK ABOUT IT, DO IT:

A lot of new moms do not like the idea of being away from their baby. Just the thought will send them into a panic. Arrange a sitter and plan the date. Make it for a couple of hours and within a few minutes of home. Tell her you're going on a date and then go…

Some date ideas include:

- Running errands she needs to get done (it makes it not a chore)
- Taking a walk together
- Scheduling a couple's massage
- Hanging out at a bookstore together
- Sharing a quiet cup of coffee
- Having dessert at your favorite restaurant
- Grabbing a fast (or slow) lunch
- Having a fast (or slow) dinner
- Shopping for shoes with her (if she's not up for clothing shopping)

Since the center of attention is the baby, it's easy to forget to be a couple. It takes effort to stay connected. A little effort will mean so much to her. She might resist a little, but once she breaks free she'll love you for it.

THE BOTTOM LINE:

She'll know you really love her when getting lucky doesn't mean sleeping with her—it means spending time with her for the rest of your life.

Tip #103
Your Tip and Story Go Here

As you continue on your journey through the expectant father and new dad experience, please share tips and stories that will help others anticipate, embrace, and manage the changes to come. The goal is to create the most valuable resource to help men (and their partners) navigate the expectant father process. Please visit www.DadsPregnant.com to share your tips and stories. I will be updating the book regularly to reflect the voices of our generation of pregnancy pioneers. From your most memorable accidental asshole moment to the things you wish I had included in the book, please send it my way for consideration in future editions of this book.

Thank you!
Harlan Cohen

RESOURCES

WEBSITES WORTH CHECKING OUT

When doing searches for medical information, make sure you are getting information from a trusted source. My criteria of a trusted source is one that has been medically reviewed and contains current information.

FACEBOOK GROUPS

Facebook is an amazing resource. It can be helpful for you or your partner. If you're not on Facebook, sign up for an account and investigate key groups. You will be surprised how easy it is to connect with people who are dealing with similar issues. This is particularly valuable for your partner. Please join the Dad's

Pregnant Facebook Fan group and I will include a list of valuable resources, tips, and information.

GENERAL INFORMATION
Medline Plus: www.nlm.nih.gov/medlineplus/
Centers for Disease Control: www.cdc.gov
National Institutes of Health: www.nih.gov
American Academy of Pediatrics: www.aap.org
The National Women's Health Information Center:
    http://www.4women.gov/pregnancy/
WebMD: www.webmd.com
The Mayo Clinic: www.mayoclinic.com
The Baby Center: www.babycenter.com
About.com: http://pregnancy.about.com
iVillage.com: www.iVillage.com
Dad's Pregnant Home: www.DadsPregnant.com

BIRTH LOCATION
Birthing Centers—American Association of
    Childbearing Centers: www.birthcenters.org
Homebirth: American College of Nurse-Midwives:
    www.midwife.org

BIRTH TEAM
American Academy of Family Physicians:
    www.aafp.org
American College of Obstetricians & Gynecologists:
    www.acog.org
Doulas of North America: www.dona.org
Doula Network: www.doulanetwork.com

Midwives Alliance of North America: www.mana.org
American College of Nurse-Midwives:
    www.midwife.org
North American Registry of Midwives:
    www.narm.org

BREASTFEEDING / NURSING
LaLeche League International:
    www.lalecheleague.org
American Academy of Pediatrics:
    www.aap.org/healthtopics/breastfeeding.cfm
The International Lactation Consultants Association:
    www.ilca.org

CHILDBIRTH EDUCATION
Your Local Hospital's website
American Academy of Husband-Coached Childbirth:
    www.bradleybirth.com
Lamaze International: www.lamaze.org
American Red Cross (Infant CPR / Choking):
    www.redcross.org
CPR: www.depts.washington.edu/learncpr/
    infantcpr.html

COMMON COMPLICATIONS
CDC / Centers for Disease Control: www.cdc.gov
    (search keywords)
Diabetes / American Diabetes Association:
    www.diabetes.org

Gestational Hypertension / Preeclampsia Foundation:
www.preeclampsia.org
Hepatitis B / Hepatitis B foundation: www.hepb.org
Preterm Labor / The March of Dimes:
www.marchofdimes.com

DEPRESSION
Mental Health America: www.nmha.org
National Institutes of Mental Health:
www.nimh.nih.gov
Postpartum Support International:
www.postpartum.net

FOOD SAFETY
Federal Department of Agriculture (FDA):
www.cfsan.fda.gov/~pregnant/pregnant.html
FDA (for women and childcare providers):
www.foodsafety.gov/~fsg/women.html

PRENATAL TESTING / COMPLICATIONS AT BIRTH
Chicago Center for Jewish Genetic Disorders:
www.jewishgeneticscenter.org
Cystic Fibrosis Foundation: www.cff.org
March of Dimes: www.marchofdimes.com
National Library of Medicine's Genetic Reference
site: http://ghr.nlm.nih.gov
National Down Syndrome Society: www.ndss.org
National Tay-Sachs and Allied Diseases:
www.ntsad.org

Sickle Cell Disease Association of America:
www.sicklecelldisease.org

PATERNITY LEAVE
Department of Labor: www.dol.gov/esa/whd/fmla/
National Partnership for Women & Families:
www.nationalpartnership.org
Families & Work Institute: www.familiesandwork.org

PREGNANCY LOSS
March of Dimes: www.marchofdimes.com

CORD BLOOD STORAGE
Public: National Marrow Donor Program:
www.marrow.org
Private: Umbilical Cord Blood Education:
www.parentsguidecordblood.com

MATERNITY CLOTHES
Gap Maternity: www.gap.com
Old Navy Maternity: www.oldnavy.com
Ann Taylor Loft Maternity:
www.anntaylorloft.com/maternity
Mimi Maternity: www.mimimaternity.com
Motherhood Maternity: www.motherhood.com
A Pea in the Pod: www.apeainthepod.com

SHOPPING FOR BABY
The Baby Bargains Book: www.babybargains.com

PARENTING HELP
The Happiest Baby on the Block:
www.thehappiestbaby.com

RECOMMENDED READING:

Solve Your Child's Sleep Problems: New, Revised, and Expanded Edition—by Richard Ferber, M.D.

Baby Bargains, 7th Edition: Secrets to Saving 20% to 50% on baby furniture, gear, clothes, toys, maternity wear and much more!—by Denise and Alan Fields

The Happiest Baby on the Block: The New Way to Calm Crying and Help Your Newborn Baby Sleep Longer—by Harvey Karp, M.D.

Mayo Clinic Guide to a Healthy Pregnancy—Mayo Clinic

Pregnancy Blues: What Every Woman Needs to Know about Depression During Pregnancy—by Shaila Kulkarni Misri, M.D.

The No-Cry Sleep Solution: Gentle Ways to Help Your Baby Sleep Through the Night—by Elizabeth Pantley

Child of Mine: Feeding with Love and Good Sense—by Ellyn Satter

The Vaccine Book: Making the Right Decision for Your Child—by Robert Sears, M.D.

Healthy Sleep Habits, Happy Child—by Marc Weissbluth, M.D.

EXPECTANT DAD'S DICTIONARY

As an expectant father, you'll come across words and expressions that aren't all that familiar to you. To help, we've indexed all the keywords (see index) and I've written a song you can sing during the ride to the hospital (or birthing facility). This is sung to the tune of Supercalifragilisticexpialidocious (from Mary Poppins). You can hear the live recorded version of this song and check out the Expectant Dad's Dictionary by visiting www.DadsPregnant.com.

Expectantfathersdosomuchbutnoonethinksaboutus
(sung to the tune of Supercalifragilisticexpialidocious)

The layette's newborn clothing, epidurals numb her pain
A registered nurse midwife's like a doctor—not the same
Doulas do the coaching and lamaze class helps her breathe
Episiotomies will make the perineum bleed

That perineum's skin between her buttocks and her crotch
If baby's too big they will cut and she will say, "Ouch"
But if she's drugged and numbed, an epidural in her spine
The pain will be more tolerable, and ohhh she'll feel so fine

Expectantfathersdosomuchbutnoonethinksaboutus...
If we say it loud enough, they'll curse us out and cuss us
Expectantfathersdosomuchbutnoonethinksaboutus...
If we say it loud enough, they'll curse us out and cuss us

The cervix, that's the opening to her uterus
When it dilates 10 centimeters—almost time to push
But first it must efface, that's when the cervix gets sooooo thin
AND then it's time for pushing, let the screaming now begin

Three stages of labor and delivery, that's what she will go through
Stage one: labor and transition, pushing, that's number two
Cut the cord and say hello—but wait there's still stage three
The placenta and the afterbirth comes, then you'll shout with glee

Choose a water birth or home birth (please cover up the floor)
A natural birth means that she'll leave pain killers at the door
Medically-assisted births can leave her numb below the waist
A C-section means the baby will come from a different place

Expectantfathersdosomuchbutnoonethinksaboutus…
If we say it loud enough, they'll curse us out and cuss us
Expectantfathersdosomuchbutnoonethinksaboutus…
If we say it loud enough, they'll curse us out and cuss us

Big engorged breasts spritz and spray, leaking happens too
Clogged milk ducts can cause mastitis, an infection, yep it's true
Stitches, bleeding, hemorrhoids from delivery they can linger
When applying hemorrhoid cream and witch hazel gladly lend a finger

No sex, sleep deprivation, colicky baby crying on your lap
It seems so rough, but it's not tough, that's if you take a nap
But when you look in baby's eyes, you'll see what that love can do
Just wait a year and then you'll be expecting number two!

HARLAN CAN SPEAK AT YOUR EVENT

Harlan has been entertaining and informing audiences for over a decade with his keynotes, events, and workshops. Harlan can customize a program to fit the needs of your group or organization at conferences, conventions, and seminars.

Topics Harlan addresses:

GENERAL AUDIENCES

- **Preg-Man-See:** A Never Before Seen Look at The Expectant Father Experience
- **Dad's Pregnant Too!:** An Expectant Couple's Guide to The Expectant Parent Experience

- **Dad's Pregnant Too! For Moms:** What Every Mom-to-Be Needs to Know about Her Man

FOR CAREGIVERS
- **Dad's Pregnant Too!:** What Expectant Fathers Want, Expect & Need From Caregivers

ADDITIONAL KEYNOTES & PROGRAMS

Based on Harlan's bestselling book (*The Naked Roommate*) and syndicated advice column (Help Me, Harlan!).

- **Training for the Sport of Taking Risks:** How to Always Win, Regardless of the Score
- **Dating in the Nude:** The Secret Truth to Finding a Date (while sober)
- **Why Smart People Do Stupid Things:** A Guide to Being Smart when Being Stupid
- **The Naked Roommate:** And Everything Else You Might Run Into in College
- **Your Kid's Naked Roommate:** And Everything Else Your Student Will Run Into in College

For more information on Harlan's events please visit him at www.DadsPregnant.com or www.Help MeHarlan.com

ABOUT THE AUTHOR

Harlan Cohen is a nationally syndicated advice columnist, bestselling author, speaker, and singer/songwriter.

Harlan's writing career started at Indiana University's school newspaper, the *Indiana Daily Student*. He shifted his path toward advice after interning at *The Tonight Show with Jay Leno* in the summer of 1995. Harlan came up with the idea to write his column after speaking with a writer who had penned an advice column in college. Upon returning to IU, he immediately launched his Help Me, Harlan! column. At first, he wrote questions and answers to himself (he helped himself), then the "real" letters started arriving. He consulted experts on and off campus to help with his replies. This delicate mix of honest advice, valuable resources, and a touch of humor turned the column into an instant success on campus. Like a bad rash at a nudist camp, Harlan's column soon spread throughout the country and beyond.

Harlan is the best selling author of *The Naked Roommate: And 107 Other Issues You Might Run Into in College* (Sourcebooks) and *Campus Life Exposed: Advice from the Inside* (Petersons). He is a contributor to *Chicken Soup for the Teenage Soul III*, an occasional contributor to the *Chicago Tribune*, and has written a monthly column for the Classroom Edition of the *Wall Street Journal*. His expert advice has been featured in *Psychology Today*, the *New York Times*, and *Seventeen* magazine. When not writing books and advice, Harlan can be found speaking across the country, appearing on radio and TV, writing and performing music from his new album, *Fortunate Accidents*, and expanding his Web sites (www.HelpMeHarlan.com, www.TheNakedRoommate.com, www.DadsPregnant.com). He is the founder of Rejection Awareness Week (RAW) and the president of the International Risk-Taking Project. His Help Me Harlan! advice column is distributed by King Features Syndicate.

Harlan lives in Chicago, IL, with his pregnant wife, daughter, and dog.

INDEX

C

caffeine 38

cancers, ovarian 466

carbon monoxide detector 302

Centers for Disease Control (CDC) 411

certified nurse-midwife 18, 22

cervix 46, 48, 54, 66, 72, 100, 122, 190, 268, 276, 356, 384, 393, 400–404, 413–14

    dilates 402

    incompetent 67, 69

checkup, annual 60

Chicago Center for Jewish Genetic Disorders 66

child, healthy 79

Child Welfare Information Gateway 162

childbirth

    education 359

    embraced 360

chiropractor 20

chlamydia 429–30

chorionic villus sampling (CVS) 63, 65

chromosomal abnormalities 59

circumcision 29, 369, 371

class

    infant CPR 353–54

    parenting 447, 450

    prenatal 224

conception 3–4, 83–84, 106

condition

    baby's 429

    cervical 268

    preexisting 25

congenital

    heart problems 59

    hypothyroidism 431

consultant, lactation 24, 350, 463–64, 468

Consumer Product Safety Commission (CPSC) 301–302

contact, skin-to-skin 426–28

contraction monitor 142

contractions

    counting 140, 357, 395

cord blood

    banking 364

    donation 368

    storage 28–29

    units 367

cramping 75, 171, 193–96, 268

cramps

    abdominal 73

episiotomies 19, 23, 350, 400, 402, 407, 491

estrogen 91, 168, 177, 208, 490

exam
    7-week 58
    abdominal ultrasound 74
    GUYne 45, 362

expectant fathers
    educated 121

expectant mother 18

F

false labor
    contractions 100

Family and Medical Leave Act (FMLA) 344

family
    bed 371, 477
    history 364, 366

father
    adoptive 161, 163
    biological 160–63
    first-time 382

FDA 331

feeding
    infant 433
    nighttime 236, 476
    weeknight 476

fertilized egg 84
    implants 3, 74

fetal monitors, electronic 407–408

fetus 38, 63, 65, 72, 74, 89–90, 270, 331

fluid, amniotic 65, 94, 99, 168, 184, 190

folic acid 37

formula feeding 371

G

gastrointestinal tract 187

Gaucher's disease 60

gender
    baby's 56, 302

genetic
    birth defects 63
    counseling 62
    counselor 62, 66
    disorders 60–61, 63

genital area 416

gonorrhea 429–30

grandparents 47, 288, 312, 354, 474, 476

grief counselor 80

group health
    benefits 29
    plans 29–30

gynecologist 14, 46

H

hair
  dyes 250
  vellus 92
hand breast pumps 465
hand sanitizer 395
hazards, choking 303
HBV 431
hCG 3, 65, 85
headaches 73, 146, 171, 234
health coverage 30
health insurance
  plan 247
  providers 25, 28, 343,
    391
Health Maintenance
  Organization 30
heart
  defects 64
  palpitations 234
heart rate
  baby's 314, 407–408
  increased 169
hemorrhaging 380
hemorrhoids 170, 189–90,
  262
hepatitis 431
herbal tea 39
HG (Hyperemesis
  gravidarum) 71–72

hormonal changes 52, 170,
  210, 325
hospital
  birth 20–21, 23
  forms 368
  paperwork/medical 340
human chorionic
  gonadotropin 65
hydrotherapy 359
hyper-ventilation 234

I

immunizations 370
infant
  CPR 352, 354
  mortality 455
  nail clippers 287
  potty training 336
  seat 245, 306, 308
infants
  calming reflex 454
  choking 354
  helping 467
infection
  newborn eye 429
instincts
  man's 391
  paternal 369, 448
  woman's 391
insurance
  agent 25

HAPPILY EVER AFTER...

Life is 90 percent amazing and 10 percent difficult.

Too often the 10 percent can take up 100 percent of our time if we're not prepared for it. The more we can understand the 10 percent, the less time it will consume.

And that's a happier, healthier, and better balanced life.